Industry Endorsements for:

The Business of Show Business

"Cynthia Brian is a true benchmark for excellence and honesty in this industry. Her enthusiasm and drive is infectious. Just watch any of her TV shows—where else can you get straight forward, up to date information without the usual little "white lies"? I've known her for many years, and not once has she dodged a question or not solved a problem. She is always charming, vibrant and filled to the brim with positive energies (which I think she must receive directly from the stars!). I am not the only one who wished she could be a part of my family."

—Norbert Brein-Kozakewycz, photographer

*"There are so many services and training opportunities out there for actors, and given most actors don't have the time or money to try them all, having a resource like "**The Business of Show Business**" is vital. You can "meet" the best in the business because host and author, Cynthia Brian does the research for you. In addition to being entertaining, you get answers to the questions about approach, philosophy, goals, location — things you would ask if you were there."*

—Sue Walden, Founder, Improvworks

"Cynthia Brian is one of the rising stars in the television world. I expect to see her picture in a feature piece right alongside Oprah and Rosie in the very near future. She exudes a life and energy that is simply irresistible"

—Stewart Heller, Executive Producer of the Emmy Awards, National Academy of Television Arts and Sciences, San Francisco/Northern California Chapter

"Cynthia Brian is a gem! Her professionalism is beyond compare! Would I work with Cynthia at the nearest opportunity? Heck yes!"

—Kathy McGraw, actor

*"I feel **The Business of Show Business** is an invaluable tool for people who are interested in starting a career in acting and modeling. Cynthia offers easy to understand information on finding an agent. The industry is plagued by people who are trying to take advantage of those who are less informed. I am so excited that Cynthia is reaching out to all of those people."*

—Bonny Eiffert , Former Commercial Print Agent, Stars, the Agency

"*The Business of Show Business* has all the steps in one sensational medium. All the info you need in one fabulous series.. The book and the show are a necessity for anyone thinking of a "showbiz" career. Cynthia Brian is a top notch professional whose creative spirit and industry knowledge inspire her readers, viewers and talent at all levels. The Business of Show Business is driven by a 'cut to the chase attitude'. In a word...brilliant!"

—**Susan McCollom**, voice-over coach, Voiceworks

"*How lucky we are that Cynthia Brian has put together* **The Business of Show Business**. *Since this industry has the worldwide allure and mystique that it does, it is so easy for people's dreams to be smashed with false hopes as well as having their finances eaten away by disingenuous people and less than honest companies. Cynthia has managed to answer any question someone might have about this business we call show.*"

—**Marie J. Salerno**, Business Coach, former Associate Executive Director AFTRA/SAG San Francisco

"*The Business of Show Business* is to actors and models what scissors and brushes are to hair stylists and make-up artists...ESSENTIAL! This book is your toolbox for success. Buy it!"

—**Denise Johnson**, Media and Commercial Hair and Make-up Artist

The Business of Show Business

A Comprehensive Career Guide for Actors and Models

Cynthia Brian

Foreword by
Richard Nelson Bolles

13th Edition

STAR★STYLE ®
Moraga, California

Published by:
Starstyle® Productions
P.O. Box 422
Moraga, California 94556

http://www.star-style.com

A portion of the proceeds of The Business of Show Business will be donated to the charity, Be the Star You Are!, a 501 (c) (3) whose mission is to empower youth at risk and raise their self esteem. Please visit: http://www.bethestaryouare.org for more information.

Warning and Disclaimer:

This is an informational guide on acting, modeling, and the entertainment industry. It is sold with the understanding that the author and publisher are not engaged in rendering legal, financial, or tax advice. Please consult with legal and accounting professional for these needs.

Every effort has been made to make this manual as accurate and complete as possible. The entertainment industry is a rapidly evolving business and therefore some content information may have changed by the time you read this. This guide is informational and educational only and does not offer any guarantees of success or work in the fields of acting and modeling. The author and publisher shall bear neither liability nor responsibility to any person or entity with respect to any loss or damage caused, or alleged to have been caused, directly or indirectly, by the information contained in this edition.

You may return this book to the publisher for a full refund if you do not want to be bound by the criteria noted above.

Starstyle® is a registered trademark of Cynthia Brian
13th edition
Printed in the United States of America

LCCN 2002091956
ISBN, printed edition 0-9721140-0-9
ISBN, PDF edition 0-9721140-1-7

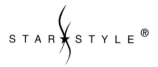

STAR STYLE ®

Contents

Acknowledgments

So many people have crossed my path in life and I am very grateful for their wisdom and support. Most of all I want to thank my parents, Al and Alice Abruzzini, who always told me I was the greatest and encouraged me to follow my heart, no matter where it lead. My love to my husband, Dr. Brian Sheaff, who has witnessed and endured the many ups and downs of our industry with me. It is rare to keep a marriage together in this business, but somehow we have muddled through the twists and turns and kept our eyes on the prize…our family unit! Our children, Justin and Heather, have been my daily inspiration and my greatest achievement in life. Both kids have worked with me in the entertainment field and their college education has been financed by their acting jobs. Although by the age of 12 Justin decided he'd rather pursue my father's passion and be a farmer, rancher, and firefighter, Heather has continued to thrive in her acting and modeling career. Today she and I work together on projects on a regular basis and it is my ultimate joy to share the spotlight with her. One day I hope to be in the audience when she receives an Academy Award! I am so proud of you both as you are both living your passions and pursuing your dreams. That is the most important aspect of living.

My greatest appreciation and gratitude to Richard Nelson Bolles, best selling author for over 30 years of "What Color is Your Parachute?" for writing my foreword. Mr. Bolles and I met when I interviewed him on my radio program a few years ago, and since that time we have become excellent friends and colleagues. He was the perfect person to write the foreword as he is considered the guru of job hunting. He helps millions of people around the world with his web site http// www:jobhuntersbible.com. It is probably no coincidence that my book, "The *Business of Show Business* has been called the "actor's bible" for over 18 years! Mr Bolles and I share the same mission in life… to help other people find their purpose and their special gifts. Thank you, Richard, for your love, support, friendship, and guidance throughout the years.

My appreciation to Pat Hallberg for being my proof reader as well as the amazing Literacy Outreach Coordinator for Be the Star You Are! charity. Pat is a not only a great actor, but a terrific friend and co-worker. Special thanks to Norbert, my photographer, who consistently captures me at my best in his lens and to Robert Howard for his creative design of my book. Without the constant expertise of Suzanne Ackerman, my Starstyle® web master and Kim Carlson, the Be the Star

You Are!® charity's web master, I wouldn't be able to keep the world apprised of my ongoing work. Thank you, ladies, for your hours of dedication, I am amazed at your talent. My gratitude to all the industry professionals who endorsed this book and because of their positive words have made it a best seller. May I extend my gratitude to the many people I have worked with over my two decades in this industry...agents, talent, producers, directors, casting people, crew members, union officials, photographers, suppliers, and publicity personnel for their opinions, experience, and beliefs. This book is a compendium of all that I have learned from the many faces that grace our magnificent industry. And huge hugs to all my clients, both children and adults, who have given me the privilege of coaching them. I feel I have learned so much from your energy, enthusiasm, and creative spontaneity.

Keep shining brightly. Kudos!

Cynthia Brian

Foreword

When we are young we dream of magic worlds,
Where we can play a thousand diff'rent parts,
And be now old, now young, now in between,
Amusing well or touching people's hearts.

We act, we sing, we dance, we help build sets,
This in your youth, both in our dreams and play,
And we know where we want our feet to go
When as adults, our dreams at last hold sway.

We want to conjure up familiar worlds,
Or kingdoms never ruled by mortal man,
We want our art to grow, as we spin webs
Manipulating face, and voice, and hand.

Our dream: to be on stage, and by our craft
To win the prize all show biz people seek
No, not applause, instead that silent awe
From patrons who are just too moved to speak.

So, you want to be in 'show biz,' is that it?
And now "that question" haunts you, day by day
"How do you find the path, break down the doors
Bust into show 'biz' when there seems no way?"
A guide, a guide, is what you need - - someone
Who's gone before, kept notes, writes well, loves You,
Can guide you step by step, past all pitfalls;
Knows what is bad advice, and what is true.

Her name? It's Brian….Cynthia.
She wrote this book, oh yes she did,
She wrote out ev'ry letter.
She's wonderful! So is her book.
You never will find better
Advice. It takes persistence, luck,
(You know) if you'd go far,
But she is right, you're setting out
To be the star
That you already are.

Richard N. Bolles, author,
What Color Is Your Parachute:
A Practical Manual for Job-Hunters & Career-Changers

Dedication

The Business of Show Business is dedicated with love and gratitude to my family, colleagues, and clients who are truly showbiz angels disguised as friends.

You are the STARS of my starstyle life!

Introduction

Actors are storytellers.

Throughout the ages, wise storytellers have reawakened the inner spirits of their listeners and inspired them to explore new territories. Stories allow us to dream and give us the courage to act upon our dreams. Stories help us discover and remember meaningful information. A story informs us by synthesizing complex issues, ambiguous situations, and opposing forces. Stories can challenge conventional wisdom, showing us people who deviate from traditional practices and produce breakthrough results. Actors take stories and breathe life into the characters offering insights as well as entertainment. Acting is a noble profession and we must all take great pride in working in a masterful manner.

However, just because we are experts in our field, does not mean we understand the business arena in which we must work. It is for this reason that in 1984 I wrote my first *The Business of Show Business* manual. In the early 1970's when I began in this industry, there was no one that I was aware of who could coach an actor in the business aspects. There were hundreds of books explaining "how to act", but none that could tell me how to create my acting and modeling business plan. I plunged into this career head first, no consideration for the jeopardy in which I had placed my person. I made every mistake possible, from getting expensive unnecessary head shots, to looking in the phone book for agents, listening to scam operators and not understanding the financial and tax ramifications. I learned the ropes by the seat of my pants…definitely trial and error and mostly error. It took me years to understand that show business is not only a trade but a business venture. I wrote my guide and all subsequent books to help each person who has ever dreamed of being an actor or model understand these slippery ropes.

It is with great pleasure that I submit to you the new 2002 version of Starstyle® Productions, *The Business of Show Business*. This handbook provides accurate, updated information on how to get going and stay going in the commercial, film, modeling, and television business. This handbook is directed to parents of babies, children, and teens as well as adults who are willing to tap into that child inside in order to become more vulnerable and knowledgeable, while avoiding the scams. As an acting coach and consultant, I take great pride in assisting clients to be the best that they can be. My speciality is coaching children for on-camera work while guiding their parents through the quagmire of challenges incurred in the entertainment industry.

It is my intention with this actors bible to give you updated and valid information regarding acting, agents, unions, casting, trade publications, photographers, modeling, classes, scams and much more. Because this is a rapidly changing business, contact information may have altered since publication. (With the rapidly growing market of cell phones, faxes, pagers, and the Internet, it is difficult to keep track of all the various area codes, web sites and other numbers) There are always new casting people, agents and photographers emerging, and, alas, others going out of business. In order to keep updated, you may need to refer to your phone directory, agent, web site search engine, or local acting bookstore. I am always available for phone or email consultations on an hourly fee basis to keep you informed.

Writing a book is hard work. Since the last version of this book in 1998, I have become a New York Times best selling author with *Chicken Soup for the Gardener's Soul* (HCI) and *Be the Star You Are! 99 Gifts for Living, Loving, Laughing, and Learning to Make a Difference* (Ten Speed Press/Celestial Arts). During the time I was writing those books, I continued to coach clients while being active in the entertainment world. It was so thrilling to watch my clients land major roles in television series, films, commercials, and modeling jobs. So often, I found myself feeling like a proud mother hen cackling with joy for her talented chicks! I also wrote, produced and hosted the national educational television series, *The Business of Show Business*, as well as hosted a popular personal growth radio program. In fact, after the release of the books, I was a guest on over 500 radio programs and numerous national television shows as an expert in the fields of gardening, personal growth, and of course, acting. With this knowledge and expertise acquired over two decades of work in the entertainment field, I feel profoundly capable of helping you become a better communicator so that you may achieve your thespian dreams with this new edition.

Almost everyone I have ever met wants to be an actor or thinks he/she could be an actor. Without counting actors who are members of both unions, there are over 135,000 people of Screen Actors Guild and the American Federation of Television and Radio Artists. (173,000 people if you count the total number of members of both unions). According to the American Theater Association more than 350,000 adults act every year in amateur productions... just for the fun of it. Ten times more children participate in theater activities. Many people make acting a lifelong avocation, and many would like to cross over into the realm of professional but are not sure how to go about it. Acting demands patience and commitment because there are long stretches between employment opportunities.

If I had a penny for every parent who told me that they had the most exquisite child alive, I'd be a wealthy woman. The truth is, there is only ONE perfect child in the world...and every mother has that child. That's the way it should be. As parents it is our responsibility to love, cherish, and believe in our offspring. However, when it comes to being a child star, not every child has the ability, the current'"popular" looks, or the tenacity and perseverance to make a commitment to acting as a career.

How do you know if you should get your child into this business?

Listen to your child. If he or she pesters you FOREVER about wanting to be on television or in a film you may have a pretentious possibility in your midst.

If you have the ability to look at your child objectively to assess the possibilities without getting into the "I have the most wonderful child" trap, enroll your child in a one day on camera workshop. If the child comes home ebullient and excited, get a consultation from a working acting coach who will be able to provide an unbiased professional assessment. Do not go to an advertised "modeling school" that may tell you only what you want to hear.

How do adults know if this would be a great second career?

Give it a shot, but be prepared to put in lots of hours of training, pounding the pavement and paying your dues. Like any new business, acting has some start-up costs. Often I find that getting jobs is just a matter of being "the last one standing." In other words, you have to show up over and over and over again. Rejection is the name of this game. The financial rewards can be great. They can also be disappointing. You can get established, or you can give up. Life is a choice and the choice is always yours.

What does acting have to do with everyday life? Everything! Acting reflects life and life is reflected in acting. The same techniques and exercises that I use to teach acting and self-esteem are useful for anyone in almost any situation. After reading this business bible, you may decide that a career in acting and modeling is not for you. That is one of the purposes of this book-to help you make an informed choice based on accurate information. Whatever your decision, let me encourage you to take an acting workshop or drama class just to fully experience a new methodology that could support you in other areas of your life. Life experiences are the core substance of acting.

Although many clients wish that I would represent them as their agent, I want to make it clear that I am NOT a talent agent. My goal is always to be a MENTOR to my clients and assist them in getting more work through a franchised talent agency. Because my first love is acting, and my second love is coaching, I have the unique opportunity to serve both purposes with a passion by being an actor and acting coach. Because I am not an agent, you can always be reassured that any advice you read in this book or receive through a consultation will be in YOUR best interest...not the interest of the agent, the producer, the client...just YOUR best interest.

I have experience in all areas of this business as an actor, writer, producer, director, set designer, and client, and let me tell you it is the actor that needs the most assistance. It is always the talent that gets the short end of the stick unless the talent (actor) knows exactly what he/she is doing. Don't think that just because you have an agent that the agent will look after your needs or make you a star. That rarely happens. You and only you have the ability and responsibility to make "it happen", whatever the "it" means to you.

Every talent is called an ACTOR regardless of sex. Several years ago, the Screen Actors Guild decided that it would be in the best interest of all thespians if we were all called "actors" instead of "actors and actresses". The nomenclature is confusing at some award ceremonies where a "Best Actor" and "Best Actress" award are still given. The Screen Actors Guild Awards Ceremonies, the only award presentation event voted upon by peer actors, presents a statuette called "The Actor" to all winners each spring. The awards celebrate the "Outstanding Performance by a Male Actor" and "Outstanding Performance by a Female Actor" in several categories. I like this approach, therefore, in my book, all thespians will be referred to as "actors".

The most important piece of advice to remember is that acting is a business, not a hobby. That's why we call it SHOW BUSINESS. Treat this career with the same determination that you would any new endeavor and you will be successful. Be professional, be skilled, and don't give away your talent.

It is my hope that this guide will become your actor's bible, an invaluable tool to assist you on the road to acting. I am always here to guide and serve you. I wish you great success in your endeavors to enter the world of acting for the camera. For children and adults, your sense of self-confidence, self-direction, and self-esteem will be enhanced. Tell your stories via your acting vocation, they need to be seen and heard. Best of luck and always remember:

You are the greatest!

May you enjoy abundance and success.

BE THE STAR YOU ARE®!

Cynthia Brian

Chapter 1

Cynthia Brian's
Favorite Quotes

Attitude

"The longer I live, the more I realize the impact of attitude on life. Attitude, to me, is more important than facts. It is more important than the past, than education, than money, than circumstances, than failures, than successes, than what other people think or say or do. It is more important than appearance, giftedness, or skill. It will make or break a company, a church, a home. The remarkable thing is we have a choice every day regarding the attitude we will embrace for that day. We cannot change our past...we cannot change the fact that people will act in a certain way. We cannot change the inevitable. The only thing we can do is play on the one thing we have, and that is our attitude. I am convinced that life is 10% what happens to me and 90% how I react to it. And so it is with you...we are in charge of our ATTITUDES."

Charles Swindoll

Your altitude is determined by your attitude.

"BE THE STAR YOU ARE"

BE A STAR!

You
can be
a star if
you believe
in yourself. You
may not be a big success the first time you
try anything new. Don't give up. Keep trying and
learning. Sometimes, success comes more
slowly than we would like, but some
things just take a certain
amount of time. Remember....
You can do it. Winners never,
You're OK.   never quit.
So, never   Quitters
give up.   do not
Win!   win.

Thomas Rische

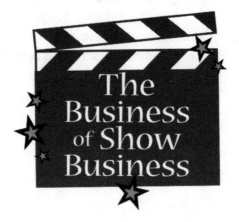

Chapter 2

On Self Esteem

"When we treat a man as he is, we make him worse than he is. When we treat him as if he already were what he potentially could be, we make him what he should be."

Goethe

We develop a sense of self relative to our surrounding world. Our self-esteem takes shape in the first three years of life. A young child's sense of self is formed through relationships with adults closest to him/her, usually parents. Since parents aren't perfect, and neither are children, most people grow up with some type of impairment to self-esteem. We can increase self-esteem at any age.

Children with high self-esteem have higher IQ's, are more effective students and learn more easily. They are healthier and happier young people. Children with low self-esteem tend to exhibit self-destructive behaviors, are disruptive and usually do poorer in school. They may become involved with alcohol or drugs, have eating disorders, run with the wrong crowd and sometimes resort to suicide. Adults greatly influence the self-esteem of children whether they intend to or not or whether they realize it or not. Through interaction with important and confident adults, children learn about their own worth. Through acting, children can learn their own individuality and a sense of their own potential. By using special techniques in visualization, imagination, creativity, and improvisation, children understand that their uniqueness is their greatest asset. It is alright to be different—in fact, being different is welcomed!

In all my workshops and consulting sessions, the special qualities of each person are examined and recognized. Children and adults are taught to take measured risks, to reach out, stretch and grow in awareness without fear of ridicule or failure. I provide a safe, supportive, and stress-free environment where each person can achieve unlimited confidence. Acting helps everyone find out who he/she is and what powers sit untouched in our mind. Many adults lack self-esteem. It is possible through the exercises of acting to recover positive aspects of character and increase esteem and self-empowerment while communicating effectively in a changing world.

Self-esteem is embodied in my slogan of *"Be the Star You Are!"* By understanding that each of us is unique and special, possessing individual talents that set us apart, we can begin to understand and celebrate our God-given gifts. We must love ourselves first, then we will automatically love others. We must learn to shout,"I am the Greatest!" and mean it. Know that we are not all going to win Emmy's, Academy Awards, or Grammy's but if we are following our heart, doing our best, and living each day to the fullest, we will experience self-esteem and personal power.

A person with healthy self-esteem is able to accept criticism, rejection, and failure while pursuing a goal. Although we may get upset, high self-esteem helps us to push aside those feelings and learn from mistakes. Take pride in things in which we excel. Acting is a business of rejection. If we can look at each "NO" as being closer to a "Yes", we will be propelled to move forward, accepting our limitations and taking comfort in our abilities. There are three attributes that all actors, young and old, need to be successful:

Perseverance, Perseverance, and Perseverance.

Everyone can reach the stars in this life

Conceive, Believe, Achieve!

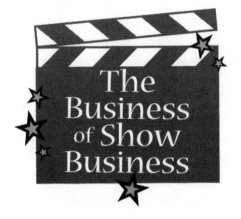

Chapter 3

Preparation for the Business

"Plan your work and work your plan."

*T*his is a competitive business, but if you are really motivated and enthusiastic about acting, you must do as much for yourself as possible. As actors, we have three tools that get us work: our mind (which is our imagination), our voice (which creates our characters) and our body (which is our motion language).

Most people have the misconception that as soon as they get an agent, their career is going to take off. WRONG! Even if you have a great agent, you can't expect an agent to be as interested in your career as you are. Therefore, although I will go into more detail later in this book, in this section, I am going to give you some "Quick Tips" to help you help yourself. Follow these simple instructions, and you'll be on your way to working in show business in record time.

Cynthia Brian's "Quick Tips"

"In the end, the only people who fail are those who did not try".

☆ Always shoot head shots with a professional "head shot" photographer. You are only as good as your photographs that look like you.

☆ Send your photo and resume out to casting directors, agency people, anyone who may be a possible work contact. Create a database of people who can hire you in the industry and keep this current. If they don't know you exist, they can't cast you in a job.

☆ Keep studying. Take workshops, do improvisation, get involved in school or community plays. Enroll in singing, dancing, martial arts, and mime classes. Do everything you can to fine tune your instrument which is your body, voice, and mind.

☆ Auditions are always stressful, but searching for the acting job is the real job of actors. The actual acting is the icing on the cake, the fun part.

☆ As much as we hate television commercials, we must watch the current commercials. Copy what the people do, mimic their lines immediately after they say them. How do you sound? Do you sound real? Do you sound as good or better than the actor on TV? Think of different ways that you could have performed the commercial. LISTEN to your voice. Is it cracking? Especially pay attention to commercials with people your age in them. How many lines did they have to memorize? Could you do that? What does their hair look like? How are they dressed? Soon, you'll start seeing a pattern forming. This is what commercials want to see in the performers they hire. If you don't look like the image portrayed on TV, you can bet you won't be hired in a similar situation.

☆ What do you look like? Maybe you'll need to consider cutting or changing your hair. Does long hair seem to be the norm, or are most girls wear a bob and boys have a beach cut? Unless you are planning on a rock video, the green mohawk probably won't do! Also, tattoos are taboo as are multiple body piercing. Use the stick on tattoos and clip on body jewels.

☆ Get a date book, day runner, planner, or palm computer to keep records of where you go, when, and who you see, and which agent sent you. Keep audition records, addresses, what to wear, what to bring, colors that will work, etc. Print out and keep this information for future use.

☆ Keep accurate records for tax purposes with receipts for everything you claim. Make sure you keep track of your mileage and write in your day runner what you are doing in the business each day. Buy a computer program, such as Quicken, for easy tracking.

☆ Buy good maps so that you can easily refer to them when you are called. In fact, buy two sets, one for your office and one for your car. Many auditions and jobs are in dangerous areas, so asking directions on the street is not recommended. You can always use the maps on the internet to plot your way. (my favorite sites are: http://www.mapquest.com or http://maps.yahoo.com) exactly where you are going before you leave and have that print out or map in your vehicle in case you get lost. Do not ask the agent or casting director for directions. They are busy and probably don't have directions from your house anyway! For work in the San Francisco area, you must have maps of San Francisco, Oakland, Marin, San Jose, and Contra Costa County and Sacramento.

☆ What's your name? In case you have decided to use a stage name, make sure you and everyone in your family knows what it is. When you go on auditions, answer the phone, make an outgoing phone message, write notes, check in with agents, or fill out registrations, use your new stage name. This is especially necessary with children who really don't understand that they are supposed to answer to a new name.

☆ Get a Social Security number and an entertainment work permit for minors under the age of 18 from your State Department of Labor Standard. In order to complete an I-9 form (which proves you are eligible to work in the United States), it is recommended to make copies of your social security card and birth certificate, passport, or driver's license. I advise carrying at least 5 copies of these documents with you at all times.

☆ Don't drop out of school or quit your job. My advice is always to have "screw you money", which translates into always having enough money to have a roof over your head, gas in your car, food on the table, and clothes on your back. In other words, you will survive if you don't get this audition. For new actors, plan on having at least 2 –3 years of earnings saved up. It could take that long or longer before you get your first pay check.

☆ Get an answering machine on your phone and order call waiting or use a reliable answering service. It is important that the agent or director can reach you the first time or there may not be a second time. They do not have the time to keep calling back on busy numbers. Most calls come during business hours but occasionally you will get evening and night calls. You want to be reachable. Make your outgoing message short without any music or children's voices. You may enjoy your selection of tunes and may think that your toddler has the cutest voice, but an agent or casting person who is trying to reach you swiftly find these messages extremely annoying. If many members of your family use the telephone frequently, you may consider installing an additional phone line to use exclusively for work. When you can not personally pick up the telephone, it is best to let the answering machine pick up. DON'T have toddlers, young children, babysitters or hearing impaired elders answer your business line. Casting people would prefer getting a message machine to talking to a child. Letting your children, babysitters and grandparents answer your business line may result in you losing the audition or job.

☆ Get a pager and/or cell phone. Almost all the current agents require talent to be on a pager or cell phone. It's best to get the area code for the major city where the jobs are as casting directors and agents often call those numbers for short notice bookings before others. (For San Francisco Bay area, ask for area code 415, in Los Angeles, get a 310, 213, 818 or 323 or area code)

☆ Know your sizes. Be prepared to fill in casting sheets with color of hair, eyes, height, weight, shoes, hat, glove, inseam, sleeve, dress, shirt, pants, bust, waist, and hips. Be accurate on your sizes. If a stylist is purchasing clothing for the shoot and you don't match the sizes that you gave to the stylist, another actor/model may be called to take your place.

☆ Look like your head shot! Keep your black and white head shots updated to look the way you look now. Children usually need new photos every year to year and half. Adults will need a new head shot every year to two years, unless a change has taken place. If you change your hair or your look, it is time to re-shoot. Your head shot is your sales kit and without a good one you won't be submitted for upcoming jobs.

☆ Keep your resume updated and remember no matter how young or new to the business, you do have a resume. Be honest and don't list extra work as if it was principal work. Staple your resume to the back of an 8 1/2" x 11" head shot.

☆ Keep your agent updated. Let your agent know if you get braces, lose teeth, break a leg, will be on vacation, or if you are unavailable for work at any time. Keep them posted on what you are doing to further your career, what plays you can be seen in, what awards you have won and any extra-curricular activities that are important. Do this by mail or postcard so that it will be kept in your file. Send them any newspaper clippings that feature you. With email, it's easy to keep in touch.

☆ Be informed. For marketing purposes, it is advised to purchase an annual copy of your local film production directory. These essential compendiums list the names, addresses, production companies and many services that you may need for your new business adventure. In Los Angeles, "The 411 Directory" is essential; in San Francisco, it's "The Reel Directory".

☆ Beware of the scams. If it sounds too good to be true, it is too good to be true. There are no free lunches. Be prepared to pay for services rendered. Remember, legitimate agents get paid by commission of your gross AFTER you have completed the job when the paycheck arrives from the client. Agents DO NOT get any fees up front.

☆ Get help. Find a reputable acting coach or consultant who can mentor you. Having someone knowledgeable, trustworthy, and active in your industry to answer the myriad of questions which are sure to appear, will save you time and money.

☆ Make a plan. Where do you want to be in five years, three years, one year, one week? How do you expect to achieve your dream? Every successful company sets goals. How will you know if you arrived, if you don't know where you are going? If you fail to plan, you plan to fail.

Should you wait to be discovered? Well, that is up to you. My advice is to seize every opportunity, be professional, get a private acting evaluation and a consultation from a pro and market your self. Get out there and pound the pavement... network, make connections and be your own best advocate.

Only <u>you</u> can make <u>you</u> a success. Go for it!
Don't give up! You have what it takes!

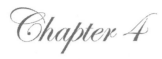 *Chapter 4*

What Kinds of Jobs Are There?

"Opportunities are usually disguised as hard work."

A brief overview of the types of work available in the acting and modeling industry. Not all cities will have agents that market these opportunities.

Modeling for Print Work

Modeling for Print Work comprises both fashion print and commercial print.

Print work is anything that is a type of modeling that is shot to be used on the printed page...magazines, newspapers, posters, billboards, point of purchase, labels, cartons, and advertisements.

☆ Fashion print for children is available for infants through teen as long as the child fits the clothing exactly. (Not the size a child will grow into, but the size that fits perfectly today) Sizes range from 3 months to 12 years.

☆ Fashion print for teens and adults requires the current "in" look, a height of a minimum 5'81/2" for women (preferably 5'9") and 5'11", 42 regular for men. Each agent specializes in a different style and will advise their fashion models accordingly.

☆ Commercial print for children and adults is plentiful and prosperous. Commercial print is anything that promotes a product, excepting clothing and cosmetics.

Rates: Print work is usually compensated by an hourly wage with the current minimum being $150.00-$200.00 per hour for adults and $125 to $150.00 per hour for children. Rates vary by location. Generally agents receive a 20% commission on the gross for print work. Vouchers are usually used instead of contracts.

Fashion Modeling and Ramp Work

Fashion models need to meet height and size requirements, usually the same as above for fashion print. Models do fashion shows and are compensated for rehearsals and per show. Some fashion shows pay by the hour.

On all print and modeling jobs, make sure to ask your agent for your rate of pay before accepting the booking. Sometimes agent negotiate "buy-outs" or a per day fee. Models are usually considered "independent contractors" and as such will be paid the full amount of the negotiated fee without withholdings less commission. A "1099" is sent at the end of the year for tax purposes by the employer or agent. It is customary to wait 30-90 days for payment of talent fees on all model jobs. There are no modeling unions as watchdogs to help with disputes, so it is up to the model to be diligent in following up for payment with the agent or client.

On-Camera and Voice Over Work

On-camera and voice-over work includes the following performing opportunities:

☆ Feature Films	☆ Radio
☆ Television	☆ PSA's
☆ Commercials	☆ CD-Rom
☆ Industrials	☆ Teaching films
☆ Voice-Overs	☆ Student Films
☆ Videos	☆ Multimedia

These categories can be either union or non-union. Principal and background work is available, with rates varying accordingly. Agents do not usually collect a commission on background work nor do they do the bookings for it.

For non-union work, rates are whatever you or your agent negotiate and can vary in length of time to make the payments to you. Agent commissions on non-union work is 20% of the gross. Stay on top of your agent or the client to assure a timely payment of the fees you negotiated.

For union rates, (our performing unions are AFTRA and SAG, discussed later in this book) please contact the union or your agent for the current rate schedule. If you are a union member, always check and double check if the program you will be working on is operated under a current valid performers union contract. It is your responsibility to do so. Working as a "scab" on non union productions can harm your reputation, your pocketbook, and your union solidarity. Don't risk it.

Agent commissions for all union work is 10% of the gross. (Please note: The Agent/Union contract is being renegotiated as this book went to print. The agent commission on union jobs may be increased. Please check with SAG or AFTRA for current regulations.) Often the contract will stipulate plus 10% which means that 10% is added to the total rate to include the agent commission. With a "plus 10%" contract, the talent does not deduct any commission from the contracted fee. In the cities of Los Angeles, Chicago, Detroit, Atlanta, Washington, D.C., and Hawaii, the contract must stipulate "scale plus 10%" for the agent to take a commission. At union scale, no commission is payable to agents in those cities.

Talent payment schedule is regulated by the unions according to the specific contract. When working under a union contract, talent is considered an employee, therefore all taxes and withholdings will be deducted from the initial payment. A W-4 must be completed at the time of work and a W-2 will be sent to the performer at the end of the year for tax purposes.

Because of the proliferation of the Internet, computers, cable and satellite companies, the growing number of independent producers and networks, there is more work than ever before for all actors in all categories.

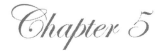

Chapter 5

Business Talk and Abbreviations

"What you think about and talk about comes about!"

*B*efore I begin telling you all about agents, audition techniques, and other acting information, it is best if you become familiar with the terms we use in this industry. Learn the lingo and you'll be sounding like a professional in no time flat.

AUDITION: Performance, usually put on video. Bring head shot.

INTERVIEW: Client is usually present to talk to you.

GO-SEE: An interview for a print job.

A CASTING: An audition or interview.

TALENT: The actor or model.

CLIENT: The person who employs the talent.

AD MAN: Representative of the advertising agency.

THE CAST: The people who got the job, principals.

YOU'RE CAST!: You got the job!

BOOKING: This means you are hired!

CALL: The job.

CATTLE CALL: An interview or audition where everyone is welcome, often known as an "open call".

CALLTIME: Time you are to report to location or audition.

CALLBACK: The second or third interview or audition for the same product or client.

CONFLICT: A commercial or job that is in direct competition with ones in which you have already performed. For example, Ford versus Chevy, MacDonalds versus Burger King

COMMISSION: A percentage paid to an agent for procuring work. For print and non-union work, the standard commission is 20% of gross. For union work, the usual commission is 10% of the gross.

ON HOLD: You are to keep free a set day and time for a job. You may have the job or are being considered. Does not guarantee a definite booking, but the client wants first priority.

LOCATION: Where the job will be shot.

THE SET: The place at the location where the shooting takes place.

THE SHOOT: The filming.

FITTING: Appointment to try on the wardrobe.

WARDROBE: Clothes you bring to the shoot.

CHANGES: Outfits worn while performing

STYLIST: The person who assists with wardrobe or set design.

MAKE-UP ARTIST: The person who applies the make-up on the shoot.

HAIR STYLIST: The person who styles hair on the shoot.

COMPOSITE: Three or more photographs on one sheet. Some may be color. Usually used for print and fashion.

HEAD SHOT: 8 1/2" x 11" black and card stock with one or two photos on it, usually a close up of head/shoulders and a 3/4 body.

ZED CARD: A 6" x 8", 5" x 7" or other size determined by agency which is used mostly for fashion modeling instead of a headshot.

TEAR SHEETS: Published work from magazines, newspapers or advertisements that can be "torn out" and placed in your portfolio.

PORTFOLIO: A compendium of photos and tearsheets to professionally display your work. Portfolios should be brought along on all auditions.

IN SIZE: Fit models who are an exact size and work doing fit modeling.

RESUME: A truthful litany of your work in film and television.

PRINT: Still photographs for newspaper or magazines.

PRINCIPAL: A role which is integral to the story. Usually a lead and entails lines.

BACKGROUND WORK: another name for being an extra.

MINOR: Any person 18 years of age or younger. Cannot work without a valid entertainment work permit.

WORK PERMIT: All children under the age of 18 must have this legal document in order to work. It is free from the California State Department of Labor Standards.

LABOR LAWS: Each state strictly enforces laws to protect children and all actors. Get a copy of the laws from the Department of Labor Standards.

PAYROLL COMPANY: The people who issue the checks!

SIGNATORY: Clients signed to a union contract.

BACK-UP BABY: Clients usually book two children on a job when they are under 5 years of age. Back up babies work 60% percent of the time. If the child is not used, usually 1/2 rate is paid.

CONFLICT: Two competitive products. In commercials you may not advertise for competitive products.

UNION: S.A.G. is Screen Actors Guild; A.F.T.R.A. is American Federation of Television and Radio Artists, and Equity is for stage.

AFL-CIO: The American Federation of Labor/Congress of Industrial Organizations.

MEMBER REPORT: A form that the performer must fill out when working under A.F.T.R.A. jurisdiction.

CONTRACT: On a S.A.G. job this is a legal employment document provided by the producer.

VOUCHER: A document for print modeling to be filled out by model and client and given to the agency.

TALENT AGENCY: Representatives of the actor/model who looks out for best interests, contracts, etc.

CASTING DIRECTOR: Employed by the production company or advertising agency to contract talent. Casting persons usually contact talent agents for a packet of head shots of available actors/models.

BOOKING OUT: When unavailable for work for any reason, you contact your agent and say you are "booking out".

I-9: Legal document which must be filled out each time of employment for a new product or film. It is necessary to prove American citizenship with two forms of identification.

TAFT HARTLEY: A waiver which permits talent to work for 30 days on a union job before they are required to join the union.

BLOCKING: The actual physical movements by actors in any scene.

BEAUTY SHOT: The shot over which credits are rolled.

AVAIL/FIRST REFUSAL: A courtesy extended by an agent to a producer indicating that a performer is available to work on a certain job. No contractual or legal status implied.

BREAKAWAY: A prop or set piece which looks solid but shatters easily, used for stunts.

DUPE: A duplicate copy of a film or tape, also called a "dub".

EMANCIPATED MINOR: A child who has been given the legal status of an adult by a judge.

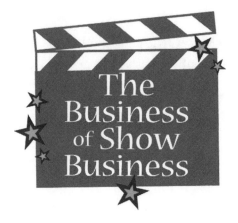

Chapter 6

The Unions: SAG and AFTRA

"Behold the turtle! He makes progress only when he sticks his neck out."

Whenever I consult with clients, the two most frequent questions asked of me are: "What is the purpose of the unions and how do I get an agent?" In this chapter, we will address the issue of unions and in the following chapter you can learn everything about agents and how to find a good one.

First of all, SAG stands for Screen Actors Guild while AFTRA stands for American Federation of Television and Radio Artists. The main purpose of both unions is to better the wages and working conditions of their members. In this respect, they negotiate the terms of contracts, length of working days, turnaround time, required school hours for minors, percentages that producer's must pay into union pension and health insurance benefits, etc. The union guarantees that payment will be made and acts on the performer's behalf when terms of the contract are breached. Neither union is an employment or placement agency. The unions also do NOT help non-members with housing, employment, or financial assistance. The unions assist with health and safety issues only on SAG/AFTRA-covered projects. The unions do NOT help anyone with connections nor can they give recommendations for the best acting schools, teachers, agents, managers, or casting directors. The unions do keep a list of current franchised talent agencies, and casting directors in the locale.

For over two decades the unions attempted to merge. Unfortunately the merger was vetoed by voting members of SAG in certain cities, therefore no merger has materialized. The unions operate independently of one another. As it stands today, actors must become members of both unions (becoming dual card holders) if they wish to work in the mediums governed by both unions. This means qualifying to join, paying initiation fees and semi-annual dues to both unions. My greatest hope is to have one strong union someday. United we stand, divided we fall.

Screen Actors Guild (SAG) has exclusive jurisdiction over principal performers in feature motion pictures and productions shot on film. SAG shares jurisdiction with AFTRA regarding television commercials, programming, and industrial/educational films.

American Federation of Television and Radio Artists (AFTRA) presides over performers in live television, radio programs and commercials, and musical recordings. AFTRA shares jurisdiction with SAG with respect to industrial/educational films, television programming and commercials.

Because of the influence of the internet and ever changing technology, there are numerous gray areas where either union may have jurisdiction. Always contact the unions for verification of your upcoming job.

The unions franchise talent agencies and union members may only work with these approved agencies. The union requires that the agent's commission be limited to 10% of the gross work under union contracts, however negotiations are in progress to increase the commission to 20% with other stipulations. Please check with the union for more details.

So how do you become a member? With AFTRA, it is easy. You fill out the forms, pay your initiation fees and dues and you are now an AFTRA member. However, as with SAG, once you join AFTRA, Rule A states that you may not work in any non union productions.

SAG is more difficult. In order to work in a SAG job you must have a SAG card, but you can't get your SAG card until you've worked in a SAG job. (The old Catch 22 dilemma!) What does one do to become a SAG actor? First of all, it is important to be a great auditioner. Employers who are signed to a union contract are called "Signatories," and every Signatory is required to give preference in hiring to qualified union performers. However, if no union member is found that fits the part, production companies may audition and hire a non-union member therefore giving them "Taft-Hartley" status. This means that the performer may work for 30 days under a union contract, enjoying all the benefits before having to join the union. My advice is this: if you are over five years old, and have the opportunity to join SAG, make sure you have enough substantial screen credits before running out to join SAG.

With so many extra players being allowed to join SAG via the "3 day loop hole", having the initials, SAG, after your name does not carry the clout that it did in by gone days. The time to join is when you are ready to make a professional commitment to the industry. If you are dedicated to staying in the San Francisco Bay Area or any small town, your work opportunities may be limited compared to those of actors who are prepared to travel to Los Angeles, New York, or Chicago. There are fewer jobs in San Francisco and other smaller communities, but there are also fewer actors in these areas, so the possibility of becoming a big fish in a small pond is a reality. Wherever you live, it is important to accumulate acting credits before making the leap to "Hollywood" where you may end up pumping gas or waiting on tables. Get some experience doing experimental or student films, and then join when you have a Taft Hartley as a principal performer.

An important matter to remember is that once you become a union member, you may not work on non-union jobs. This is called Rule 1 in SAG and Rule A in AFTRA. SAG enforces Global Rule One which means that all SAG actors must be covered by a SAG contract when working outside the United States. There are severe penalties for disobeying these rules.

How do you know if a production company is "signatory"? A good rule of thumb is to ask anyone who sticks a camera or microphone in your face if their company is covered by a union contract. This includes voicemail and interactive disc voices as well. If you are not sure, call your nearest union local.

In simplest terms, the unions are for the benefit of the actor, young and old. Until you are a union member, you are not considered a professional in the industry. Virtually every television show, film and commercial you will ever see employs union talent. The union gets us higher wages, better working conditions, per diems, travel and wardrobe expenses, a health, pension, and retirement plan, credit union, and great food on shoots. Most important of all, it keeps track of and sends us our residual payments for all work done. I'm still getting several checks a year from my first film, "Raid on Entebbe" with Charles Bronson which I made in 1976. The residuals may be small, but it is like finding money on the street! I'll take it gladly and gratefully. These checks alone have paid for my dues over the years!

When working under SAG or AFTRA contracts, the performer is never an independent contractor as is the case most often with modeling or non-union work. Under Guild Agreements, performers are employees for all purposes and compensation is subject to all appropriate payroll taxes, and deductions such as FICA, Medicare, FIT, SDI, and State income tax. Performers must complete W-4's at the beginning of employment and earnings should be reported on W2 forms at the end of each calendar year.

Whenever in doubt about any union audition or job, contact your local union office. The people are there to serve the members. Staff are happy to take your calls and answer your questions. The unions will always be your best advocates.

Spotlight on Screen Actors Guild

Screen Actors Guild, (AFL-CIO) also known as SAG, is chartered as part of the Associated Actors and Artistes of America (the Four A's) which includes the American Federation of Television and Radio Artists (AFTRA), Actors' Equity Association (AEA), the American Guild of Musical Artists (AGMA), and the American Guild of Variety Artists (AGVA). SAG is also a member of the International Federation of Actors (FIA) which is a global organization of performer's unions. SAG represents approximately 98,000 professional actors and performing artists nationally working in feature films, television, commercials, industrial and educational videos, student and experimental films, and music videos.

Members work as principal performers, stunt performers, singers, dancers, voice-over performers, pilots, puppeteers, extras, and models. Age range is newborn to over 100 years old. Unfortunately, 85% of SAG members earn less that $5,000 per year, with only about 5% earning above $50,000. Of course, the big stars earn millions!

Hollywood and the Los Angeles area boast the largest number of SAG members with New York, Florida, Chicago, and San Francisco in second through fifth places. There are branches of the union, often combined with AFTRA, across the United States.

SAG does not secure employment for its members. The Guild's primary responsibilities include negotiating contracts which establish minimum wages and working conditions, enforcement of those contracts, processing residual payments, regulation and franchising of talent agents, membership record-keeping and communications. SAG is also concerned with the general welfare and quality of living of its members. There is excellent medical coverage for those who qualify by earnings as well as a pension plan.

Joining SAG:

As of July 1, 2002, the initiation fee to join is $1310, plus the basic minimum semi-annual dues of $42.50. The National initiation fee is calculated at twice the current theatrical/television day player rate which is currently $655, to be $678 beginning July 1, 2003. There are rates for weekly performers, singers, dancers, stunt performers and TV series actors. SAG general extra players receive $110 per day going up to $115 on July 1, 2003. SAG dues are based on earnings and are billed twice per year. Each SAG member will pay a basic $85.00 dues annually. Members earning more than $5,000 per year under SAG contracts will pay 1 1/2% more in dues to a maximum of $150,000. Members who are paying full dues to another performer's union and earn less than $25,000 per year under SAG contracts receive a $10.00 reduction in dues per year. Members whose SAG earnings exceed $25,000 pay full dues, regardless of other guild affiliations.

A performer may become eligible for SAG membership under one of the following conditions:

1. Proof of SAG employment as a principal player under a SAG contract from a signatory company. Proof of employment is required which may be the signed contract, payroll check or letter from the signatory company. Documentation must include social security number, name of production, salary paid and dates worked.

2. Proof of SAG employment as an extra player under a SAG contract for a minimum of three work days. Proof of employment and documentation are the same as above.

3. If an applicant is a paid-up member of an affiliated performers' union (AFTRA, AEA, AGVA, AGMA, or ACTRA) for a period of one year and has worked as a principal performer in that union's jurisdiction at least once.

Appointments are necessary before going into a SAG office. All applications are fully investigated for validity and any false statements will jeopardize chances to join the union and may be subject to disciplinary proceedings.

RATES:

There are many variables in session fees. For current information on rates it is best to contact your local SAG office or visit the web site at http://www.sag.org. The following is a general description for current minimum day rates as of this writing.

FILM:

☆ For principal work in a feature film, the current SAG day player rate is $655.

☆ For SAG extra work in a feature film, the rate based on an eight hour day is $110.

COMMERCIALS:

(The commercial contract is a joint AFTRA/SAG contract.)

> ☆ For commercial work, the current on-camera principal performer rate is $500.
>
> ☆ For off-camera principal performer is $375.95
>
> ☆ For hand models unlimited use rate is $419.70
>
> ☆ For extra performer unlimited use is $275.

Please check with the union before accepting any employment to discuss the appropriate fees and residual possibilities.

RULE ONE:

Once a performer joins SAG, that performer is prohibited from working in any non-union project or for any producer who has not signed the collective bargaining agreement with the Guild. There is no such thing as a "waiver" to work in a non-union project. GLOBAL RULE ONE makes it the right and responsibility of the actor to ask for and receive a SAG contract for all performances outside of the United States. Global Rule One is a very high priority for the future security of the Guild and its members.

WEBSITE:

Updated information is always available at
http://www.sag.org

Spotlight on AFTRA

AFTRA is a chartered local of the American Federation of Television and Radio Artists, AFL-CIO. The National AFTRA is chartered as part of the Associated Actors and Artistes of America (the Four A's), which also includes Actors' Equity Association, the American Guild of Musical Artists, the American Guild of Variety Artists and Screen Actors Guild.

Nationally AFTRA represents approximately 75,000 broadcasters, actors, singers, dancers, announcers, newspersons, sportscasters, disc jockeys, writers, editors, directors and technicians working in television, radio, commercials, industrial and educational videos, cable and phonograph recordings.

AFTRA is a national federation of over 39 autonomous local unions located across the country. San Francisco is the fourth largest local.

The primary responsibilities of AFTRA include negotiating contracts which establish minimum wage scales and working conditions for its members with enforcement of those contracts; processing session payments and residuals, regulation and franchising of talent agents, membership record-keeping and communication. Like SAG, AFTRA does not try to find work for its members.

AFTRA also provides an excellent medical and dental plan with life insurance and a pension plan established through collective bargaining with employers.

JOINING AFTRA:

The current initiation fee to join AFTRA is $1200 with dues paid semi-annually based on income. Minimum dues payment is $58.00 A performer may join AFTRA by making an appointment, coming into the office, completing the application (allow an hour) and paying the full initiation fee plus semi-annual dues. If a performer elects to join before securing a union job, he or she must also sign an acknowledgement of AFTRA's advice that no work guarantee or access to membership in another 4-A's union is automatically provided through this membership.

RATES:

Each medium has a different base rate. Before accepting employment, contact the union to find out what the minimum scale is for your particular project. Make sure you know what the project is (CD-Rom, radio, informercial, industrial, commercial, TV show, etc.), how long it will be and where it is planned to air (cable, regional, national network, etc.) The television contract shares jurisdiction with SAG. For commercials, an on-camera principal performer earns $500, off-camera principal earns $375.95, unlimited use hand model earns $419.70.20, and unlimited use extra performer earns $275. Other rates apply for singers, dancers, groups, speakers, and foreign language commercials.

RULE A:

AFTRA enforces RULE A which stipulates that an AFTRA member may not accept employment from any employer not signatory to the union. As with SAG, non-union waivers are nonexistent.

WEBSITE:

Updated information is always available at http://www.aftra.com

Addresses of SAG Offices

SAG website: http://www.sag.org

National Headquarters:

HOLLYWOOD
5757 Wilshire Boulevard
Los Angeles, Ca. 90036-3600
323-954-1600
fax 323-549-6603

BRANCHES

ARIZONA
1616 E. Indian School Road #330
Phoenix, Arizona 85016
602-265-2712
fax 602-264-7571

BOSTON
11 Beacon Street #512
Boston, MA 02108
617-742-2688
fax 617-742-4904

CLEVELAND
1030 Euclid Avenue, #429
Cleveland, Ohio 44115
216-579-9305
fax 216-781-2257

CHICAGO
1 East Erie Street #650
Chicago, Illinois 60611
312-573-8081
fax 312-573-0318

COLORADO
950 South Cherry Street #502
Denver, Colorado 80246
800-527-7517 or 303-757-6226
fax 303-757-1769
(also covers New Mexico & Utah)

DETROIT
27770 Franklin Road
Southfield, Michigan 48034-5386
248-355-3105
fax 248-355-2879

FLORIDA (Miami)
7300 North Kendall Drive #620
Miami, Florida 33156
305-670-7677
fax 305-670-1813
(also covers Alabama, Arkansas,
Louisiana, Mississippi, South
Carolina, West Virginia, US Virgin
Islands and the Caribbean.)

HAWAII
949 Kapiolani Blvd. #105
Honolulu, Hawaii 96814
808-596-0388
fax 808-593-2636

LAS VEGAS
3900 Paradise Road, #162
Las Vegas, Nevada 89109
702-737-8818
fax 702-737-8851

DALLAS
6060 N. Central Expressway
Suite # 302 LB 604
Dallas, Texas 75206
214-363-8300
fax 214-363-5386

GEORGIA
455 E. Paces Ferry Road NE#334
Atlanta, Georgia 30305
404-239-0131
fax 404-239-0137

FLORIDA (Central)
646 West Colonial Drive
Orlando, Florida 32804-7342
407-649-3100
fax 407-649-7222

HOUSTON
2400 Augusta Dr. #264
Houston, Texas 77057
713-972-1806
fax 713-780-0261

MINNEAPOLIS/ST. PAUL
708 North First Street, #333
Minneapolis, Minnesota 55401
612-371-9120
fax 612-371-9119

NASHVILLE
1108 17th Avenue South
Nashville, Tennessee 37212
615-327-2944
fax 615-329-2803

NORTH CAROLINA
311 North Second St. #2
Wilmington, North Carolina 28401
910-762-1889
fax 910-762-0881

PORTLAND
3030 S. W. Moody #104
Portland, Oregon 97201
503-579-9600
fax:503-279-9603

ST. LOUIS
1310 Papin Street #103
St. Louis, Missouri 63103
314-231-8410
fax 314-231-8412

SAN FRANCISCO
350 Sansome St. #900
San Francisco, Ca. 94104
415-391-7510
fax 415-391-1108

WASHINTON, D.C./BALTIMORE
4340 East West Highway, #204
Bethesda, Maryland 20814
301-657-2560
fax 301-656-3615

NEW YORK
1515 Broadway, 44th floor
New York, New York 10036
212-944-1030
fax 212-944-6774

PHILADELPHIA
230 South Broad Street. #500
Philadelphia, Pennsylvania
19102
215-545-3150 fax 215-732-0086

PUERTO RICO
530 Ponce de Leon Avenue #312
San Juan, Puerto Rico 00901
787-289-7832 ext. 3212

SAN DIEGO
7827 Convoy Court #307
San Diego, Ca. 92111
858-278-7695
fax 858-278-2505

SEATTLE
4000 Aurora Ave. N #102
Seattle, Washington 98103
206-270-0493
fax 206-282-7073

Addresses of AFTRA Locals And Chapters

A.F.T.R.A. WEBSITE: http://www.aftra.com

National Offices:

New York
260 Madison Avenue
New York, NY 10016-2402
Tel: 212-532-0800
Fax: 212-532-2242
aftrany@aftra.com

Los Angeles
5757 Wilshire Blvd., 9th Floor
Los Angeles, CA 90036-3689
Tel: 323-634-8100
Fax: 323-634-8194
losangeles@aftra.com

Local and Chapter Offices:

ATLANTA
455 East Paces Ferry Rd. NE
Atlanta, Georgia 30305
404-239-0131
fax 404-239-0137
atlanta@aftra.com

BOSTON
11 Beacon Street #512
Boston, Massachusetts 02108
617-742-2688
fax 617-742-4904
boston@aftra.com

BUFFALO
2077 Elmwood Avenue
Buffalo, New York 14207
716-874-4989
c/o WIVB-TV

CHICAGO
One East Erie #650
Chicago, Illinois 60601
312-573-8081
fax 312-573-0318
chicago@aftra.com

CLEVELAND
1468 West 9th Street#720
Cleveland, Ohio 44113
216-781-2255
fax 216-781-2257
cleveland@aftra.com

DALLAS/FT.WORTH
6060 N. Cent. Expressway #302
Dallas, Texas 75206
214-363-8300
fax 214-363-5386
dallas@aftra.com

DETROIT
27770 Franklin Road
Southfield, Michigan 480346
248-355-3105
fax 248-355-2879
detroit@aftra.com

DENVER
950 South Cherry Street, #502
Denver, Colorado 80222
303-757-6226
fax 303-757-1769
denver@aftra.com

HAWAII
260 Madison Avenue
New York, New York 10016
866-634-8100 (toll free)
hawaii@aftra.com

KANSAS CITY
4000 Baltimore, 2nd floor
Kansas City, Missouri 64111
816-753-4557
Fax 816-753-1234
kansascity@aftra.com

MIAMI
20401 N. W. 2nd Ave. #102
Miami, Florida 33169
305-652-4824/4846
fax 305-652-2885
miami@aftra.com

DETROIT BROADCAST DIV.
260 Madison Ave, 7th floor
New York, New York 10016
212-532-0800
fax 212-532-2242

FRESNO
4831 East Shields Ave. #32
Fresno, California 93724
559-252-1655

HOUSTON
2400 Augusta #264
Houston, Texas 77057
713-972-1806
fax 713-780-0261
houston@aftra.com

LOS ANGELES
5757 Wilshire Blvd. 9th floor
Los Angeles, California 90036
323-634-8100
fax 323-634-8246
losangeles@aftra.com

NASHVILLE
1108 17th Avenue South
Nashville, Tennessee 37212
615-327-2944
fax 615-329-2803
nashville@aftra.com

NEW ORLEANS
2400 Augusta Drive #262
Houston, Texas 77057
877-236-2941 (toll free)
713-972-1806
fax 713-780-0261
neworleans@aftra.com

NEW YORK
260 Madison Ave. 7th floor
New York, New York 10016
212-532-0800
fax 212-545-1238
aftrany@aftra.com

OMAHA
3000 Farnham St. #3 East
Omaha, Nebraska 68131
402-346-8384

PEORIA
260 Madison Ave.
New York, New York 10016
800-638-6796 (toll free)

PHILADELPHIA
230 South Broad Street #500
Philadelphia, Pennsylvania 19102
215-732-0507
fax 215-732-0086
philadelphia@aftra.com

PHOENIX
1616 E.Indian School Rd. #330
Phoenix Arizona, 85016
602-265-2712
fax 602-264-7571
phoenix@aftra.com

PITTSBURGH
625 Stanwix Street, penthouse
Pittsburgh, Pennsylvania 15222
412-281-6767
fax 412-281-2444
pittsburgh@aftra.com

PORTLAND
3030 S. W. Moody #104
Portland, Oregon 97201
503-279-9600
fax 503-279-9603
portland@aftra.com

ROCHESTER
260 Madison Ave.
New York, New York 10016
716-467-7982

SACRAMENTO/STOCKTON
8145 La Riviera Drive
Sacramento, Calif. 95826
916-387-5129
fax 916-387-8383

SAN DIEGO
7827 Convoy Court #400
San Diego, California 92111
858- 278-7695
fax 858-278-2505
sd@aftra.com

SAN FRANCISCO
350 Sansome Street #900
San Francisco, California 94104
415-391-7510
fax 415-391-1108
sf@aftra.com

SCHENECTADY/ALBANY
170 Ray Avenue
Schenectady, New York 12304
518-374-5915
fax 518-346-6249

SEATTLE
4000 Aurora Ave. #102
Seattle, Washington 98103
206-282-2506
fax 206-282-7073
seattle@aftra.com

ST. LOUIS
1310 Papin #103
St. Louis, MO 63103
314-231-8410
fax 314-231-8412
stlouis@aftra.com

WASHINGTON/BALTIMORE
4340 East West Highway #204
Bethseda, MD 20814
301-657-2560
fax 301-656-3615
wash_balt@aftra.com

TRI-STATE
128 East 6th Street #802
Cincinnati, Ohio 45202
513-579-8668
fax 513-579-1617
tristate@aftra.com

MINNEAPOLIS/ST. PAUL
708 North First Street #333A
Minneapolis, Minnesota 55401
612-371-9120
fax 612-371-9119
wincities@aftra.com

Who's Getting Those SAG Union Roles?

"Keep climbing until you reach the star of your dreams."

Back in the early 1980's when I first started coaching other people about this business, I would begin each consultation with the current statistics on who was getting the most jobs. At that time, boys and men accounted for 75% of all principal SAG jobs. By the early 1990's, women had moved up a bit and were receiving 30% of all the roles. By 2000, women were being cast in 38% of the roles, however, women make up the majority of the population of America. According to the SAG Casting Data Reports which are based on information provided by producers to the Guild, men are cast twice as much as women and work twice as many days. Employment statistics for 2000 indicated that the percentage of roles played by SAG's women, minorities, and seniors continue to rise slowly, but at rates that do not reflect the growth and significance of these citizens.

The under 40 crowd is still grabbing the majority of the roles with a solid two out of three jobs. Women over the age of 40 were cast in only 26.2% of the roles for women, compared to 72.3% of the roles cast for women who were under the age of 40. Furthermore, leading women over the age of 40 comprised only around 20% of the roles for women in 2000. In 2000, the number of jobs jumped 7% from 49,662 in 1999 to 53,134, but women and minorities are still under represented on television and on film.

An averaged breakdown of all roles for both men and women as of 2000 is as follows:

Asian/Pacifics	2.6%
Latino/Hispanics	4.9%
African Americans	14.8%
Caucasians	77.4%
Native Americans	.30%

Ethnicity

SAG's casting data indicates that 22.9% of the roles in 2000 went to performers of color, the highest percentage since the Guild began collecting these statistics in 1992, up from the 21.2% of roles received in 1999. A total of 11,930 roles went to African Americans, Latinos/Hispanics, Asian/Pacific Islanders, or Native American Indians in 2000. These numbers indicate only the number of roles, not the importance of the roles. The populations of the United

States represents 11.4% Latino/Hispanic, so the 4.9% of acting roles is considerably lower than the populations.

The same holds true for Asian/Pacific Islanders, who reached their highest ever percentage of roles, 2.6%, but still lag behind their approximately 4.0% representation in the U.S. population.

As actors, we must keep demanding more equality in roles. The Guild is committed to increasing job opportunities for the entire membership by sponsoring events and directories directed towards those empowered to hire actors.

Nevertheless, $1.66 billion was earned under SAG contracts in 1999.

Income was generated in the following categories:

Television shows	$599.5 million
Feature Films	$423.5 million
SAG extras	$ 68.1 million
Commercials	$627.3 million
Industrials	$ 12.2 million
Residuals	$673.5 million

Based on these figures, as actors, we have a very healthy outlook for our union and for the future. This is good news for those of you who are just joining us. Let's hope your work will be included in future statistics!

Exhibit E Union sign in sheets

Audition sign in forms for commercials are called Exhibit E's. Traditionally talent signs in their name, social security number, agent, time in, actual call time, time out, # of call backs, and initials. Because the concern over unauthorized acquisition of a performer's credit information has been raised, the Guild advises using your union number on all sign in sheets. I advise not using your social security number on any document until work has been procured. This precaution is for the protection of all talent.

Exhibit E (example)

Name:	Social Secutiry	Agent:	Actual Call:	Time In:	Time Out:
Cynthia Brian	Xxxxxxxxxxx	Starstyle	2 pm	1:45pm	2:30pm
Heather Brittany	xxxxxxxxxxx	Starstyle	2:30pm	2:15pm	3:50pm

(In this example, Heather Brittany would be entitled to 20 minutes of compensation as she spent one hour and 20 minutes at the audition, whereas Cynthia is entitled to no compensation having spent only 30 minutes auditioning.)

It is important to remember to sign in and sign out. On every union audition, a performer donates one hour of time. If the audition runs over one hour, the performer is usually entitled to compensation. These forms are sent to the union office after a casting call, but only members who filled in the blanks appropriately can expect to be paid for extra time. Time begins from the time of your actual call time assuming you arrived on time, until you clock out. If you arrive early, your time would still begin at your call time. If you arrive later than your actual call time, you risk not being auditioned for the job. If you do get to audition, your time begins when you arrive and ends an hour after that. It is important to always sign in on the Exhibit E registration form.

SAG/AFTRA Member Report

All members of SAG and AFTRA are required to fill out a member report at the end of each union freelance job. The member report is a legal document and the basis for ensuring payment. Reports are obtained through the union offices. Make sure to always have enough of the various types of reports on hand for every job. Although each report will vary slightly depending on whether it is for commercials, TV, industrials, radio, etc., the basic information is similar. It is imperative that the employer or signator signs the report. After giving a copy to the signator, the member is responsible for sending a copy to the union and retaining a personal copy for records. Member reports are available from the SAG/AFTRA office. If a member has difficulty understanding the document, a call to the SAG/AFTRA office will remedy the situation.

Instructions for completing and filing a member report:

☆ It is best to print.

☆ AFTRA or SAG: make sure to check the appropriate box at the top of the joint member report.

☆ Date of engagement: This is the session date, the date you actually performed the work. Fill out a separate member report for each date.

☆ Signator or Ad Agency: Print the name and contact information for the person or company that hired you. Make sure the company that is signed to the AFTRA/SAG contract signs in all the appropriate places.

☆ Social Security Number: you must write in your social security number so that you can be compensated for your work. This is mandatory here.

☆ Sponsor and Product: This is the client, the service, or the product that is advertised.

☆ Fee to be Paid by: This is not the agent or payroll company, but the employer who hired you which would be the Signator or Ad agency

☆ Fee and 10% over scale: If you know what the session fee is, write it in the box. If it is union scale, you can write "scale". If the employer has agreed to pay you 10% over scale to compensate agency fees, check that box as well and write in the name and address of your agent.

☆ Group Reports: If there are several union actors on one job, all can be listed on one report. However it is vital to designate one actor to be responsible for getting the report to the union. It is always best to ask for a personal copy for your records.

Remember that this report is an invoice to the employer. The clearer and more detailed you are, the easier it will be for the union to get you paid on time.

Runaway Production and Right-to-Work States

For several years now, SAG and AFTRA actors have experienced a significant drop in acting roles because of producers taking their projects to other countries, especially Canada and Eastern Europe where it is less expensive for them to make their films, commercials, and TV shows. Many countries offer inviting financial subsidies to attract the entertainment industry to their shores. This problem has become known in our industry as "run away production". Both AFTRA and SAG have been working diligently to keep our productions here in the United States where American artists and citizens can benefit. Together with the United States Film Alliance, which is an association of entertainment guilds including the Directors Guild of America and other trade organizations, AFTRA and SAG are supporting federal legislation from Congress that would grant wage based tax credits and financial incentives for programs produced in the United States. Millions of dollars of revenue is spent in other countries each year as a result of the "run away productions". The goal is to encourage producers to produce in America and stop the current flow to the other side of the border. With SAG's Global Rule One in place for union actors, the diligence of all entertainment unions and some federal support, actors, writers, directors, and other artisans hope to see more work and more revenue here at home.

When you hear the phrase "right-to-work", what is really being said is "anti-union." Both guilds are dedicated to improving the working conditions, salaries, health and welfare benefits of the actors and broadcasters they serve. Many states are still anti-union and do not want their actors organized or represented by the guilds. Negotiation sessions with management to bring guild representation to the workers is available whenever the workers ask for it. So don't be fooled into thinking that a "right-to-work" area is a good thing. It is not! Be diligent and find out what union affiliations and contracts are available before accepting any job offer.

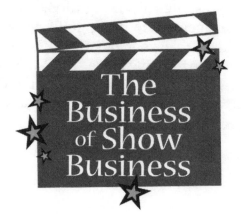

Chapter 7

Agents.....Do You Need Them?

"There are no limits except those you create for yourself."

*Y*ES, YES, and YES! In order to be considered professional and legitimate it is imperative to have an agent. In fact, without an agent, you will probably only be considered for extra work. Producers and casting people do not have time to know all the talent in the area so they rely on reputable talent agents to assist them in submitting the appropriate actors for a shoot. With the hundreds of jobs being cast in the area, without an agent, it would be difficult, if not impossible to know about or be considered to audition for such projects.

What are agents? Agents represent a variety of talent for work in commercials, print, film, fashion, voice-overs, and industrials. First of all, remember this is a BUSINESS, not a hobby. Because agents are paid on a commission basis (20% of your gross for non-union and print work, 10% of your gross if you are union, although the unions are renegotiating this amount with agents currently, so expect an increase), they expect you to be professional and business-like. You hire the agent, not the other way around, so don't be intimidated by agents. Good agents work hard for their talent by developing working relationships with producers, casting directors, creative and broadcast directors, so that their talent may be considered and cast for specific jobs. Agents negotiate fees and contracts and sometimes assist their represented talent with choosing the correct head shots. Agents expect their talent to get good training but may not tell them with whom to study or take workshops. Talent must practice their craft and learn to market themselves and work as a team with their agent. Talent must get professional 8 1/2 x 11 black and white head shots for commercial/print work and color zeds for fashion/print. (Be aware that the original print that comes from the photographer is an 8 x 10, but when it is duplicated into multiple head shots, these photos need to be made in 8 1/2 x 11 format...think paper size!)

Most agents require that a talent be exclusive to that agent which means that talent may have only one agent. The positive thing about having more than one agent is that you may be seen differently by the agents and thus submitted for more job opportunities. The negative is that both agents may submit you for the same casting, making it necessary for the casting director to choose between one agent or another which they do not like to do.

Agents are necessary and a vital, valid mainstay of our industry. Work with them, trust them, share ideas, but don't bug them. They have work to do getting us all acting jobs!

Facts About Talent Agencies

I am often asked: "How do I find a legitimate agency and how do I know they won't rip me off?"

Good question and there are some helpful answers. A legitimate agency" does not charge a fee payable in advance for registering for representation. Legitimate agencies make their money from commissions which are a percentage of your gross, which is paid to them after you have earnings. Nothing is paid in advance. Talent agencies are required to be licensed in the State of California as Talent Agents. Most of the best agents are franchised by Screen Actors Guild and the American Federation of Television and Radio Artists. Agents who have a formal relationship to the unions agree to a code of conduct negotiated between the union and the talent agency. For example, there is a limit on the amount of commission an agent can take, there are rules for contracts between agents and talent, and there are a series of protections for both agents and performers. Agency agreements with the unions are currently under review and revamping as it has been over four decades since the last neogtiation. Much has changed in those years so we can expect some revisions in the near future that will affect all performers. The unions always put the needs of the members first so we can be assured that when any new rules or regulations are implemented, agents franchised by SAG and AFTRA will be more protective of the performer.

Talent agencies franchised through the unions are forbidden from advertising in newspapers or magazines and may not solicit you through the mail. Scam agencies, on the other hand, almost always advertise and solicit through newspapers, magazines, radio ads, fairs, pageants, talent shows, and schools. Beware and be a wary consumer. Remember what I said earlier, if it sounds too good to be true, it probably is.

Legitimate talent agents also may not charge you for classes, photographs, public relations services, screen tests, acting workshops or other services. They may recommend a variety of photographers, hair stylists, make-up artists, etc., but they may not demand that you frequent a particular person for any service. If an agent that you are considering is pushing you to sign on the dotted line or go to a certain salon....run and keep your checkbook with you.

Although I have known a few good agents who were not franchised by the unions, over time these agencies went out of business or did become franchised if they were a serious agency. Before signing any contract with an agency, it is safer to make sure that agent is franchised by the unions. However, the unions have NO jurisdiction over print work, modeling or fashion, so you are on your own in this occasion. It is best to contact a trustworthy consultant or ask model friends for a referral. Looking through the yellow pages just doesn't cut it in the agency department! Any improper conduct by an agent should be reported to SAG immediately. Complaints can also be handled by the Consumer Protection division of the Federal Trade Commission. Business and personal managers are not regulated by the unions or by the state. Again, established legitimate firms don't advertise for business nor do they usually handle newcomers. Beware! Become fully informed about your rights as a consumer and the various aspects of the entertainment industry before you make any financial commitments to any enterprise. To obtain information as to the legitimacy of certain businesses, you may call the consumer action unit of the District Attorney's Office for the county in which the business is located, the

Better Business Bureau for that region, or the California Commissioner's office in San Francisco. From the Department of Industrial Relations you can request a copy of the bulletin on minors in the entertainment industry or to learn whether an agency is operating with a valid State license by calling 415-975-2065.

There is no way to know for sure if you will be ripped off, but by being a knowledgeable consumer of show business, the odds are in your favor that you'll find a good agent.

How to get an Agent

Since agents can not solicit for talent, how will you get an agent? There are three normal and acceptable ways:

1. Be introduced through a friend who already is represented by this agent or be referred by a casting person or producer.

2. Invite the agent to a play or production in which you have a lead role and hope that the agent is pleasantly impressed with your work and wants to represent you.

3. Find out which agents are franchised by SAG and AFTRA. Send these agents a short cover letter requesting representation along with a resume with your current 8 1/2 x 11 black and white head shot and a self addressed stamped envelope for a return answer. Don't send out photographs that you want returned, as agents are busy and don't have time to sort through the mail to determine what needs to be re turned. Make sure you have included a phone number where you are reachable. Expect to wait two to eight weeks for an answer.

Most actors get their agents by using scenario # 3. It is risky and time consuming for the agents to develop new talent. Agents are careful about only representing talent that they feel are bookable at this time. This doesn't mean if you are rejected by one agent, that another agent won't want you. Keep submitting until you find an agent who is willing to give you a personal interview. When you do get an interview, remember that appearance and good grooming are very important. You only have one opportunity to make a first impression. Hair, face, clothes and shoes must be clean and appropriate. Beauty is not that essential. What is important is your personality and high energy looks that come from being healthy and happy. Look like the photograph you sent in the mail. You were called in because of your look on the picture, make sure that photo represents the you NOW, not the you you used to be. Also, do not expect agents to incurr any expenses for you. All the materials you will need to present yourself as a professional are your responsibility, including your photographs, resumes, and demo reels.

Be on time. Bring with you any pertinent information that you want the agent to see. For example, contact sheets, a portfolio of work, a video of clips of movies or commercials you have done. Do not bring in family snapshots, a video of a recital or production. Any questions you want to ask the agent should be written down so that you don't waste valuable time. This is a business. Treat it as one. Be courteous, professional, friendly...but to the point. State your purpose, then leave. Be prepared to answer the most asked question in the business: "Tell me about yourself." Be passionate and succinct.

Wear clothing that makes you feel comfortable. Do not be too dressy. Do not wear jeans and a T-shirt. Do not try to look sexy. Look professional, casual, and commercial-like. You want the agent to be thinking about projects to cast you in, not where you purchased your clothes.

Once the agent has agreed to represent you, don't sit back and wait for the phone to ring. You have to take responsibility for your own career. Be informed. Get into workshops, sharpen your skills. Be prepared. Also, write the agent a short thank you note. All too often we forget to show our appreciation. Always maintain an attitude of gratitude.

What to Expect From any Agent

In order to be successful, you will need to have a good working relationship with your agent. You work as a team. Many actors are under the impression that once an agent is secured, that the actors' work is finished and that the agent will do it all. NOT TRUE! It is essential for the actor to market voraciously and to keep in contact with the agent. Promote yourself and let your agent know what you are doing to further your career. Get into plays, take classes, improve your vocal skills. If you should be contacted directly from a casting person or producer for a job, call your agent and have your agent negotiate the deal. Your agent wants you to work and it does not matter who found the job. Having your agent negotiate for you usually gets you bigger fees. I once was booked on a print job for three hours that I had anticipated charging my usual $200 per hour. When I asked my agent what she had negotiated, she said $2500 for the three hours! Obviously I was delighted and surprised. This was a definite indication of the power of the negotiating skills of my agent.

The first few months of your relationship with your agent are crucial. It is during this time that the agent is deciding if you are serious about this craft as a business or as a hobby. Agents are carefully watching your audition skills. They are interested in finding out where your niche is and how they can help you succeed. Timing is important...submitting the right actor, for the right role at the right time.

Since there are so many questions regarding an actor or model's responsibilities with agents, below is a general checklist. Be aware that each agent will work a little differently and that once you are represented by an agent, find out that agency's requirements.

General Talent Information

1. There is no fee for joining a legitimate agency.

2. Most agents will require you to be exclusive. This means you can have only one agent for print, one agent for commercials, one agent for film. Sometimes one agency will want you to be exclusive in all these departments. Some times an agency will want you only for print or only for commercials in which case you are free to find another agency to represent you in that area. Be clear with your agent. Ask your agency in what areas they will be representing you.

3. The most important marketing tool for promoting your talent is a current photo. Casting directors and clients request photos prior to scheduling an audition or go-see. Sometimes, talent will be booked directly from photos without an interview. Most agents require that you give them 25-50 photos to have on file with resumes if you are doing film and commercial work. Snapshots are acceptable for babies, but anyone over the age of 18 months needs a

professional head shot. Photographic styles change, but currently 3/4 body shots and head shots(which are head and shoulders) in black and white are used throughout the industry. For fashion, color zeds are the norm. If you are just starting, go with a black and white until you have had some paid bookings. Your agent or acting coach can suggest several professional photographers and duplicators. Plan on shooting a new head shot at least once a year.

4. Supply a statistic sheet to your agent and keep this updated. A sample statistic sheet is listed under Casting Sheet example in this book. This statistic sheet is a reference card so that your agent can quickly access your current age, sizes, phone numbers, address, etc. It is best to attach a small 2" x 2" snapshot of this sheet for their records. It is imperative to keep the agent up dated. Any change in size or looks can mean a job...for example if you get braces, break an arm, cut your hair, etc. etc. Agents are not mind readers, put it in writing. For children, size means the actual size they are wearing today, not the size they will grow into.

5. Everyone who works must have a social security number. Your agent will want to have this on file. However, do not give this number out on auditions, go-sees or interviews. Protect your privacy.

6. Anyone under the age of 18 must have a valid work permit. Information regarding the work permit is located in this book under Information for Minors. Provide your agent with a current

copy of the work permit and don't forget to update it every six months.

7. Often agents will get calls for"real families". If your family members, including pets, are willing to work with you on a job, supply your agent with a few snapshots or good color copies of your family and pets together in one shot. (Keep in mind all minors will need a work permit)

8. If you are given an agency contract, please read it carefully before signing. If you have any questions, ask your agent for more information. A parent or guardian's signature is required on all documents when the child is under 18 years of age.

9. If you will be doing modeling or print work, ask your agent for VOUCHERS. These are used for billing for print jobs. Keep these with you in your day timer or portfolio. At the end of a shoot make sure to fill it out completely and have the client sign it. Vouchers usually have 4 copies, the white is for the client, the yellow and pink goes to the agency, and the goldenrod is for your records. NO VOUCHER...NO PAY! Keep your copy.

10. Resumes should either be printed on the back of the head shot or stapled in all four corners with the information facing outward. Keep resumes updated. Do not hand an agent a stack of resumes to be stapled on the photos. The job of the talent is to do this.

11. Absolutely essential is having an answering machine with call waiting on your telephone. Some agents require you to carry a pager or cell phone at all times. You must be reachable. Little advance warning of jobs is normal and the job will be given to someone else if you cannot be reached the first time.

12. Checking in and booking out. In general, call and check in with your agent once a week or once every two weeks. Acceptable times are from 10am to noon and 2pm to 4pm. Do not call between noon and two unless it is an emergency. Many agents use this time to eat at their desks and to get organized. If you will be on vacation, or you are ill, contact your agent and BOOK OUT. Give your agent the days you will be gone. When you return, contact your agent and BOOK IN. A good way to keep in contact with your agent is by email. Ask your agent about using this easy option.

13. MAPS-get good maps and use them. As previously discussed, agents and casting people will not give you directions. Carry city maps in your car and keep an extra set at home. Always allows enough time to get to auditions and jobs. Plan for flat tires, traffic, and road construction delays.

14. Working with the client is a delicate balancing act. If you cannot make your interview for any reason, contact your agent. If you are late for a job, contact your agent, not the client directly. If you have any questions about anything, it is always best to check with your agent, not with

the client. Do not sign any contracts on a job without an agent approval, excepting of course, AFTRA and SAG contracts for work. In other words, your agent is always the middle person.

15. Never, never take extra people with you on an audition or a shoot. This is a professional "no no". Extra kids, friends, grandparents, spouses, etc. are not welcome. The rule with taking children on a job or audition is one parent or guardian allowed per child.

16. Talent can be held financially responsible to the production company for lateness, misrepresen tation, or any other misconduct. Be punctual, prepared, be professional. There is no excuse for lateness.

17. Always bring head shots and resumes on all auditions. A portfolio may be requested for print go-see's. Keep a stack in your car for peace of mind.

18. Payment schedules differ by agency. In general, paychecks are issued after the agency has received payment from the client. A 20% commission or agency fee is deducted from gross pay for all print and non-union jobs while a 10% commission or agency fee is de ducted for union bookings. If sixty days elapse and you have not received your payment, contact your agent immediately and discuss the options of getting paid. You may need to contact the client, but first check with your agent.

19. Keep excellent records of all jobs, auditions, commissions paid, vouchers, and pay stubs. Do not throw these away, ever!

20. Your success depends on your tenacity, perseverance, and business acumen. You must be committed to the development of your career and be a partner with your agent in promoting and marketing your talents and abilities. Break a leg!

Franchised Agents in the United States

Franchised Agents

Please remember only these agents, and no others are authorized to act on behalf of AFTRA members in AFTRA's jurisdiction.

If you have any questions or concerns, please call the National Agency Department at 212-532-0800. They are there to help you.

All contact information is current as of publication of this book. Please double check addresses before sending out materials as this is a rapidly changing business.

The symbols, which appear next to the agent's address, indicate the type of representation offered by that agent:

(A)	Athletes	(Mu)	Musical Artists
(B)	Broadcasters	(O)	Older People
(Ch)	Children	(R)	Phonograph Recordings
(C)	Commercials	(S)	Specialty Acts
(D)	Dancers	(T)	Television Programs
(F)	Foreign/Ethnic	(V)	Voice Over
(If)	Infomercials	(*)	People w/ Disabilities
(CD)	CD - Roms	(In)	Interactive
(P)	Promo's	(NB)	Non-Broadcast
(Id)	Industrials	(M)	Models

ATLANTA AGENTS

ATLANTA MODELS & TALENT INC.
2970 Peachtree Rd. NW, #660
Atlanta, GA 30305
(404) 261-9627
M,C,V,If,Ch,O,F,*,T,CD,It,NB,Id,P

BORDEN & ASSOC., TED
P.O. Box 11590
Atlanta, GA 30355
(404) 266-0664
A,B,CH,D,M,MU,O,S,C,R,T,V

THE BURNS AGENCY
3800 Bretton Woods Road
Decatur, GA 30032
Attn: Carrie Miller

DONNA SUMMER AGENCY
8950 Laurel Way, Suite 200
Alpharetta, GA 30202
(770) 518-9855

GENESIS MODEL & TALENT
1465 Northside Dr., #120
Atlanta, GA 30318
(404) 350-9212
M,C,V,If,Ch,O,F,*,T,CD,It,NB,Id

KELLY KELLY ENTERPRISES, INC.
10945 State Bridge Road, PMB 401-316
Alpharetta, GA 30328
(770) 446-9781
B,F,C,V,If,T,NB,Id

GLYN KENNEDY, Inc.
975 Hunterhill Drive
Rosewell, GA 30075
(678) 461-4444
M.B,A,C,V,Ch.O,F,*,T,NB,Id

TALENT GROUP/HOT SHOT KIDS
561 West Pike Street
Lawrenceville, GA 30045
(678) 215-1500
V,M,B,T,R,C,Ch,O,F,*,S

THE PEOPLE STORE
2004 Rockledge Rd., N.E.
Atlanta, GA 30324
(404) 874-6448
M,C,V,B,R,If,Ch,O,F,*,T,CD,It,NB,Id,P

THE VOICE CASTING NETWORK
8950 Laurel Way, Ste. 100
Alpaharetta, GA 30302
V

WILSON INC., ARLENE
887 West Marietta St., #N-101
Atlanta, GA 30318
 (404) 876-8555
M,C,V,If,Ch,O,F,*,S,T,CD,It,NB,Id,P

BOSTON AGENTS

ACTUAL TALENT
1260 New Britain Rd. Suite 65
West Hartford, CT 06110
Phone: (860) 920-5322
Fax: (860) 561-2473
Ch, C, F, If, CD, P, Id, O, R, T, V, NB, M

MAGGIE INC.
35 Newbury Street, 5th Fl.
Boston, MA 02116-3105
(617) 536-2639
M,F,*,C,If,T,CD,NB,Id,P

MODELS GROUP
374 Congress St., #305
Boston, MA 02110
(617) 426-4711

MODELS INC.
218 Newbury Street, 2nd Floor
Boston, MA 02116
(617)437-6212
M,A,Ch,O,F,*,C,If,T,CD,NB,Id,P

CHICAGO AGENTS

AMBASSADOR TALENT AGENTS, INC.
333 N. Michigan Ave., #910
Chicago, IL 60601
 (312) 641-3491

ARIA MODEL & TALENT MGMT., LLC.
1017 W. Washington, Suite 2C
Chicago, IL 60607
(312) 243-9400

BAKER & ROWLEY TALENT AGENCY, INC.
1347 West Washington, Suite 5C
Chicago, IL 60607
 (773) 252-7900
All Areas - Except Broadcast

BIG MOUTH
Talent Agency
935 West Chestnut, Suite 415
Chicago, IL 60622
(312) 421-4400
All Except - *

ETA INC.
7558 S. Chicago Ave.
Chicago, IL 60619
(312) 752-3955

FORD TALENT GROUP
641 West Lake Street, Suite 402
Chicago, IL 60661
(312) 707-9000

GEDDES AGENCY
1633 N. Halsted, #400
Chicago, IL 60614
(312) 787-8333

SHIRLEY HAMILTON INC.
333 East Ontario, Suite B
Chicago, IL 60611
(312) 787-4700

LINDA JACK TALENT
230 East Ohio, #200
Chicago, IL 60611
(312) 587-1155

JENNIFER'S TALENT UNLIMITED,
INC.
740 N. Plankinton, Suite 300
Milwaukee, Wisconsin 53203-2403
(414) 277-9440

LILY'S TALENT AGENCY
1301 West Washington, Suite B
Chicago, IL 60607
(312) 792-3456

LORENCE LTD, EMILIA
325 W. Huron #404
Chicago, IL 60610
(312) 787-2033

LORI LINS LTD.
7611 West Holmes Avenue
Greenfield, WI 53220
(414) 282-3500

NAKED VOICES, INC.
865 North Sangamon, Suite 415
Chicago, IL 60622
(312) 563-0136

SALAZAR & NAVAS INC.
760 North Odgen #2200
Chicago, IL 60622
(312) 666-1677

SCHUCART ENTERPRISES,
NORMAN
1417 Green Bay Rd.
Highland Park, IL 60035
(708) 433-1113

STEWART TALENT MGMT., CORP.
58 West Huron
Chicago, IL 60610
312-943-3131

VOICES UNLIMITED INC.
North Fairbanks, Suite 2735
Chicago, IL 60611
(312) 832-1113

ARLENE WILSON TALENT, INC.
430 West Erie, Suite 210
Chicago, IL 60610
(312) 573-0200

ARLENE WILSON TALENT, INC.
807 North Jefferson St., 200
Milwaukee, WI 53202
(414) 283-5600

CLEVELAND AGENTS

FORD TALENT GROUP
1300 East 9th St., Suite 1640
Cleveland, OH 44114
(216) 522-1300

IMPACT MGMT. TALENT (IMI)
9700 Rockside Road, Suite 410
Cleveland, OH 44125
(216) 901-9710

DALLAS-FORTH WORTH AGENTS

CAMPBELL AGENCY, THE
3906 Lemmon Ave., #200
Dallas, TX 75219
(214) 522-8991
A,CH,F,M,O,S,*,C,T,V

COLLINS TALENT AGENCY,
MARY
2909 Cole Avenue, Suite 250
Dallas, TX 75204-1307
(214) 871-8900
C,F,O,P,T,V,*

DAWSON AGENCY INC., KIM
2710 N. Stemmons Fwy., #700 Tower
North
Dallas, TX 75207-2208
(214) 630-5161
A,CH,D,F,M,MU,O,S,*,C,R,T,V

DOUBLE TAKE TALENT AGENCY
14902 Preston Rd., #404-324
Dallas, TX 75240
(972) 404-4436
C,V,TV,R,B,Ch,O,F,*

HORNE AGENCY, THE
1576 Northwest Hgwy.
Garland, TX 75041
(972) 613-7827

IVETT STONE AGENCY
6309 N. O'Connor Rd., Suite 100
Irving, TX 75039-3510
(214) 506-9962
C,F,O,R,T,V,*

TAYLOR TALENT INC., PEGGY
1825 Market Center Bl., #320, LB37
Dallas, TX 75207
(214) 651-7884
A,CH,D,F,M,MU,O,S,*,C,R,T,V

THE TOMAS AGENCY
14275 Midway Rd., #220
Dallas, TX 75244
(972) 687-9181
ALL EXCEPT - B, A

DENVER AGENTS

DONNA BALDWIN TALENT
Historic Wheeler Block Building
2150 West 29th Avenue, #200
Denver, CO 80211
(303) 561-1199
M,B,Ch,O,F,*,S,C,V,B,If,T,CD,In,NB,Id,P

BARBIZON TALENT AGENCY
7535 E. Hampden Ave.,#108
Denver, CO 80231
 (303) 337-7954
A,B,CH,D,F,M,MU,O,S,*,C,R,T,V

VOICE CHOICE
1805 S. Bellaire St., Suite 510
Denver, CO 80222
(303) 756-9055
C,V,R,If,T,CD,It,NB,Id,P

DETROIT AGENTS

C.L.A.S.S MODELING & TALENT AGENCY
2722 E. Michigan Ave., Ste. 205
Lansing, MI 48912-4000
 (517) 482-1833
M,D,C,V,If,Ch,O,F,T,NB,Id,P

THE I GROUP, LLC
29540 Southfield Rd., #200
Southfield, MI 48076
(810)552-8842
M,D,B,C,V,R,Ch,O,F,*,S,T,NB,Id,P

PRODUCTIONS PLUS
30600 Telegraph Rd., #2156
Birmingham, MI 48025-4532
(810) 644-5566
ALL AREAS - No CD Roms

TALENT SHOP, THE
30100 Telegraph Rd.,#116
Birmingham, MI 48025
 (810) 644-4877
A, B, CH, D, F, M, O, S,*C,T,V

HOUSTON AGENTS

ACTORS ETC., INC.
2620 Fountainview, #210
Houston, TX 77057
 (713) 785-4495
M,B,Ch,O,F,S,C,V,R,If,T,CD,It,NB,Id,P

NEAL HAMIL AGENCY
7887 San Felipe, St., #204
Houston, TX 77063
 (713) 789-1335
M,Ch,O,F,C,V,B,If,T,Id,P

INTERMEDIA AGENCY
5353 W. Alabama, #222
Houston, TX 77056
 (713) 622-8282
M,A,Ch,O,C,T,Id

PASTORINI-BOSBY AGENCY
3013 Fountainview, #240
Houston, TX 77057
(713) 266-4488
M,B,Ch,O,F,C,VO,R,If,T,CD,It,NB,Id,P

WILLIAMS TALENT, INC.
13313 Southwest Freeway, Suite 194
Sugar Lane, TX 77478
 (281) 240-3145
C,V,B,If,T,NB,Id,P

YOUNG AGENCY, SHERRY
2620 Fountainview, Suite 212
Houston, TX 77057
 (713) 266-5800
M,B,C,V,R,If,Ch,O,F,S,T,CD,It,NB,Id,P

KANSAS CITY AGENTS

THE AGENCY/MODELS &
TALENT
10 East Cambridge Circle Drive
Kansas City, KS 66103
913-342-8382
M,C,V,If,Ch,O,F,T,CD,It,NB,Id,P

ENTERTAINMENT PLUS
114 A West 3rd Street
Kansas City, MO 64105
(816) 474-4778
M,D,B,A,Mu,C,V,Ch,O,T,NB,Id,P

EXPOSURE INC.
215 West 18th Street
Kansas City, MO 64108-1204
(816) 842-4494
M,B,C,V,If,Ch,O,F,*,T,CD,It,NB,Id,P

HOFFMAN INT.
6705 West 91st Street
Overland Park, KS 66212
(913) 642-1030
M,B,C,V,If,Ch,O,F,S,T,CD,It,NB,Id,P

TALENT UNLIMITED
4049 Pennsylvania Ave., #300
Kansas City, MO 64111
(816) 561-9040
ALL AREAS - no A,*,S

LOS ANGELES AGENTS

5 STAR TALENT AGENCY
2312 Janet Lee Dr.
La Crescenta, CA 91214
(818) 249-4241

ABLAZE ENTERTAINMENT, INC.
1040 N. Las Palmas Ave., Bldg. 30
Los Angeles, CA 90038
(323) 871-2202

ABRAMS ARTISTS AGENCY
9200 Sunset Blvd., #1130
Los Angeles, CA 90069
(310) 859-0625
C,T,V,M,B,R,A,O,S,D,Ch,F,Mu

ABRAMS-RUBALOFF &
LAWRENCE
8075 W. Third, #303
Los Angeles, CA 90048
(213) 935-1700
C,V,T,B,R,O,F

ACME TALENT & LITERARY
6310 San Vincente Blvd., #520
Los Angeles, CA 90048
(323) 954-2263
C,T,Ch,O,F

THE AGENCY
1800 Avenue of the Stars #400
Los Angeles, CA 90067
(310) 551-3000
T,C,Ch,O,F

AGENCY FOR THE PERFORMING
ARTS,
9200 Sunset Blvd., 9th Fl.
Los Angeles, CA 90069
(310) 273-0744
T,B

AGENCY WEST ENTERTAINMENT
(formally J.E.O.W)
6255 West Sunset Blvd., #908
Hollywood, CA 90028
 (323) 468-9470

AIMEE ENTERTAINMENT ASSOC.
15840 Ventura Blvd. #215
Encino, CA 91436
(818) 783-9115
T,O,F,Mu

AKA TALENT AGENCY
6310 San Vincente Boulevard
Los Angeles, CA 90048
(323) 965-5600

ALLEN TALENT AGENCY
P.O. Box 1498
Los Angeles, CA 90078
 (213) 605-1110
C,F,M,D,B

ALVARADO AGENCY, CARLOS
8455 Beverly Blvd., #406
Los Angeles, CA 90048
(213) 655-7978
C,V,T,Ch,O,F,Mu

AMSEL, EISENSTADT & FRAZIER,
INC.
5757 Wilshire Blvd., Ste. 510
Los Angeles, CA 90036
(323) 939-1188
T,F,A,Mu,O

ARTHUR ASSOC., LTD, IRVIN
9363 Wilshire Blvd., #212
Beverly Hills, CA 90210
(310) 278-5934
T,C,V,Mu,S,R,B

ARTISTS AGENCY
1180 S. Beverly Drive, # 301
Los Angeles CA 90035
 (310) 277-7779
T

ARTISTS GROUP, LTD.
10100 Santa Monica Blvd., #2490
Los Angeles, CA 90067
(310) 552-1100
T,O,F,Ch,*

A.S.A.
4430 Fountain Ave., #A
Hollywood, CA 90029
(323) 662-9787
C,T,R,B,M,D,A,F,V,Mu,S

ATKINS & ASSOCIATES
303 South Crescent Heights Blvd.
Los Angeles, CA 90048
(323) 658-1025

THE AUSTIN AGENCY
6715 Hollywood Bl. #204
Hollywood, CA 90028
(323) 957-4444

BADGLEY & CONNOR, INC.
9229 Sunset Blvd., #311
Los Angeles, CA 90069
(310) 278-9313
F,O,T

BAIER/KLEINMAN
INTERNATIONAL
3575 Cahuenga Blvd., W #500
Los Angeles, CA 90068
(818) 761-1001
T,F

BALDWIN TALENT, INC.
8055 W. Manchester Avenue
Playa del Rey, CA 90292
(310) 827-2422
C,T,A,V,Mu,Ch,O,F,S,*

BALL TALENT AGENCY, BOBBY
4342 Lankershim Blvd
Universal City, CA 91602
(818) 506-8188
C,T,O,F,D,Ch,S,M,V,A,R,Mu

BARON ENTERTAINMENT
5757 Wilshire Boulevard, Ste. 659
Los Angeles, CA 90036
(323) 936-7600

BAUMAN REDANTY & SHAUL
5757 Wilshire Blvd., #473
Los Angeles, CA 90036
(323) 857-6666
V,T

BENNETT AGENCY, SARA
6404 Hollywood Blvd., 316
Los Angeles, CA 90028
(323) 965-9666
C,T,O,F,Ch,*

BERZON AGENCY, MARIAN
336 E. 17th St.
Costa Mesa, CA 92627
(714) 631-5936
T,C,V,M,Ch,F,O,*

BONNIE BLACK TALENT AGENCY
5318 Wilkinson #A
Valley Village, CA 91607
(818) 753-5424
C,T,M,O,F,Ch,S

BLAKE AGENCY, THE
/'1333 Ocean Avenue
Los Angeles, Ca. 90401
(310) 899-9898

E. THOMAS BLISS & ASSOCIATES
292 LaCienega Bl., #202
Beverly Hills, CA 90211
(310) 657-4188

BRAND MODEL & TALENT
AGENCY
1520 Brookhollow Drive, #39
Santa Ana, CA 92705
(714) 850-1158

THE BRANDT COMPANY
15250 Ventura Blvd., #720
Sherman oaks, CA 91403
(818) 783-7747

BRESLER KELLY & ASSOCIATES
11500 W. Olympic Bl. #510
Los Angeles, CA 90064
(310) 479-5611
T

BARRY HAFT BROWN WEST
ARTISTS AGENCY
9056 Santa Monica Blvd. #305
W. Hollywood, CA 90069
(310) 205-6911
T,D,F,O

DON BUCHWALD & ASSOC., INC.
PACIFIC
6500 Wilshire Blvd., 22nd Floor
Los Angeles, CA 90048
(323) 655-7400
T,Ch,B,F,*

BUCHWALD TALENT GROUP, INC.
A Youth Agency
Commercial Department
6300 Wilshire Boulevard, Suite 910
Los Angeles, CA 90048
323-852-9555

Theatrical Department
6500 Wilshire Boulevard, Suite 2210
Los Angeles, CA 90048
323-852-9559

BURKETT TALENT AGENCY, INC.
27001 La Paz Rd., Ste. 418
Mission Viejo, CA 92691
 (949) 830-6300
C,V,T,B,M,Ch,F,D,O,*

BURTON AGENCY, INC.,
1450 Belfast Dr.
Los Angeles, CA 90069
(310) 288-0121
C,T,Ch,V

C' LA VIE
7507 Sunset Boulevard, # 201
Los Angeles, CA 90046
 (323) 969-0541

CAMERON & ASSOC., INC.,
BARBARA
8369 Sausalito Ave., #A
West Hills, CA 91304
(818) 888-6107
C,V,T,Ch,O,Mu,*

CAREERARTISTS, INT.
11030 Ventura Blvd., #3
Studio City, CA 91604
 (818) 980-1315
M,D,C

WILLIAM CARROLL AGENCY
139 North San Fernando Blvd., Ste. A
Burbank, CA 91502
(818) 848-9948

CASSELL-LEVY, INC.
843 N. Sycamore
Los Angeles, CA 90038
(323) 461-3971
C,V,O,F,B,S,R,A,D,Mu,*

CASTLE HILL ENTERPRISES
1101 S. Orlando Ave.
Los Angeles, CA 90035
(323) 653-3535
C,V,T,Ch,Mu,O,F,S,*

CAVALERI & ASSOC.
178 South Victory Blvd., #205
Burbank, CA 91506
(818) 955-9300
C,V,T,M,Mu,Ch,O,F,*

THE CHARLES AGENCY
11950 Ventura Bl., Ste. A
Studio City, CA 91604
(818) 761-2224

CHASIN AGENCY, THE
8899 Beverly Blvd., #716
Los Angeles, CA 90048
(310) 278-7505
T

CHATEAU BILLINGS TALENT
AGENCY
5657 Wilshire Blvd., #340
Los Angeles, CA 90036
(323) 965-5432

CHRISTOPHER GROUP, THE TORY
6381 Hollywood Blvd., Ste. 600
Hollywood, CA 90028
(323) 469-6906

CINEMA TALENT AGENCY
2609 Wyoming Ave., #. A
Burbank, CA 91505
(818) 845-3816
C,V,T,F,A,Ch,O

CIRCLE TALENT ASSOCIATES
433 N. Camden Dr., #400
Beverly Hills, CA 90210
(310) 285-1585
C,T,Ch,F,O,*

CLARK CO., W. RANDOLPH
13415 Ventura Bl. #3
Sherman Oaks, CA 91423
(818) 385-0583
C,T,Ch,O

CLER TALENT AGENCY, COLEEN
178 S. Victory Bl. #108
Burbank, CA 91502
(818) 841-7943
C,M,Ch

COAST TO COAST TALENT
GROUP, INC.
3350 Barham Blvd.
North Hollywood, CA 90068
(323) 845-9200
C,V,T,M,A,O,Ch

THE COLORING BOOK
An Artists Agcy.
650 N. Bronson Avenue
Bronson Bldg., #B144
Hollywood, CA 90004
(323) 960-4795

COLOURS MODEL & TALENT
MGMT.
8344 1/2 W. 3rd Street
Los Angeles, CA 90048
(213) 658-7072
T,C,M,Ch,O,F,R,B,V,S,*

COMMERCIALS UNLIMITED
8383 Wilshire Blvd., #850
Beverly Hills, CA 90211
(323) 655-0069
C,V,M,D,A,B,Ch,O,F

COMMERCIAL TALENT
9157 Sunset Blvd. #215
Los Angeles, CA 90069
(310) 247-1431

CONTEMPORARY ARTISTS, LTD.
1317 5th St., #200
Santa Monica, CA 90401-2210
(310) 395-1800
T,O,Ch,F

THE COPPAGE COMPANY
3500 W. Olive Ave. #1420
Burbank, CA 91423
(818) 953-4163
T

CORALIE THEATRICAL AGENCY, JR.
4789 Vineland Ave., #100
North Hollywood, CA 91602
(818) 766-9501
C,V,T,M,D,Ch,A,O,F,Mu,S

COSDEN ENT., LTD., ROBERT
7080 Hollywood Blvd. #1009
Los Angeles, CA 90028
 (213) 874-7200
T,V,C,Ch,O,Mu,F,B,A

CREATIVE ARTISTS
9830 Wilshire Blvd.
Beverly Hills, CA 90212
(310) 288-4545

THE CROFOOT GROUP, INC.
23632 Calabasas Rd., Suite 104
Calabasas, CA 91302
(818) 223-1500
T,V,B

CULBERTSON-ARGAZZI GROUP
8430 Santa Monica Blvd. #210
W. Hollywood, CA 90069
(323) 650-9454

CUNNINGHAM, ESCOTT, DIPENE
& ASSOC., Inc.
10635 Santa Monica Blvd., #130
Los Angeles, CA 90025
(310) 475-2111
ALL AREAS

DADE-SCHULTZ ASSOC.
23905 Plaza Gavilan
Valencia, CA 91355
 (818) 760-3100
T,O,F,Ch

DDK TALENT AGENCY
3800 Barham Blvd. #303
Los Angeles, CA 90068
(310)-274-9356

TALENT
1800 N. Highland, #300
Los Angeles, CA 90028
(323) 962-6643
ALL AREAS

DIVERSE TALENT GROUP
1875 Century Park East #2250
Los Angeles CA 90067
(310) 201-6565
C,V,T,Ch, O,F,*)

CRAIG DORFMAN & ASSOCIATES
9200 Sunset Blvd. #800
Los Angeles, CA 90069
(310) 858-1090

EBS/Los Angeles
3000 W. Olympic Blvd. #2438
Santa Monica, CA 90404
310-229-5989

EDWARDS & ASSOCIATES, LLC
655 North Central Avenue, 17th Floor
Glendale, CA 91203
(323) 964-0000
C,V,TV,B,Ch,M,O,F,S

ELLE CHANTE TALENT AGENCY
231 West 75th Street
Los Angeles, CA 90003
(323) 750-9490

THE ENDEAVOR AGENCY, L.L.C
9701 Wilshire blvd., 10th Fl.
Beverly Hills, CA 90212
(310) 248-2000

EPSTEIN - WYCKOFF - CORSA -
ROSS & ASSOC.
280 S. Beverly Dr., #400
Beverly Hills, CA 90212
(310) 278-7222
C,V,T,A,Ch,O,F

EVOLVE TALENT AGENCY
3435 Wilshire Boulevard, Suite 2700
Los Angeles, CA 90010
(213) 251-1734
(All)

FERRAR MEDIA ASSOC.
8430 Santa Monica Blvd., #220
Los Angeles, CA 90069
(323) 654-2601
C

FILM ARTISTS ASSOC.
13563 Ventura Blvd., Fl 2
Sherman Oaks, CA 91423
(818) 386-9669
ALL AREAS

FLICK EAST-WEST TALENT, INC.
9057 Nemo St.
West Hollywood, CA 90069
(310) 271-9111
C,T,M,OF

FONTAINE AGENCY,
205 South Beverly Dr., #212
Beverly Hills, CA 90212
(310) 471-8631
C,M,O,Ch

FREED COMPANY, BARRY
2040 Ave. of the Stars #400
Los Angeles, CA 90067
(310) 277-1260
T

ALICE FRIES AGENCY
1927 Vista Del Mar Ave.
Los Angeles, CA 90068
(323) 464-1404
T,O,Ch,F,S,R,M,B,D,Mu,A

GAGE GROUP, INC.
9255 Sunset Blvd., #515
Los Angeles, CA 90069
(310) 859-8777
T,C,V,O,F

DALE GARRICK INT.
8831 Sunset Blvd., #402
Los Angeles, CA 90069
(310) 657-2661
C,T,B,Ch,F,O,*

GEDDES AGENCY
8430 Santa Monica Blvd., #200
West Hollywood, CA 90069
323-848-2700
T,F,*
T

HALPERN & ASSOC.
12304 Santa Monica Blvd., #104
Los Angeles, CA 90025
(310) 571-4488
T,B,M,A,O,F

HAMILBURG AGENCY,
MITCHELL J.
8671 Wilshire Bl. #500
Beverly Hills, CA 90211
 (310) 657-1501

HART & ASSOC., VAUGHN D.
8899 Beverly Blvd., #815
Los Angeles, CA 90048
(310) 273-7887
T,F,O

HECHT AGENCY, BEVERLY
12001 Ventura Pl., #320
Studio City, CA 91604-2626
(310) 505-1192
T,C,Ch,F,M,O

HENDERSON-HOGAN AGENCY
247 S. Beverly, #102
Beverly Hills, CA 90212
(310) 274-7815
F,O,*,T

HERVEY-GRIMES TALENT
AGENCY, INC.
10561 Missouri #1
Los Angeles, CA 90025
(323) 475-2010
C,T,O,Ch,M,F,*

HOLLANDER TALENT GROUP
14011 Ventura Blvd. #202W
Sherman Oaks, CA 91423
(323) 845-4160
C,V,T,Ch

HOUSE OF REPRESENTATIVES
TALENT
400 S. Beverly , #101
Beverly Hills, CA 90212
(310) 772-0772
T,F,O

HOWARD TALENT WEST
11374 Ventura Bl.
Studio City, CA 91604
(818) 766-5300
C,T,Ch,O,F,*

 HWA TALENT REPRESENTATIVES
3500 W. Olive Avenue #1400
Burbank, CA 91505
(818) 972-4310
T

IFA TALENT AGENCY
8730 Sunset Blvd. #490
W. Hollywood, CA 90069
(310) 659-5522

INNOVATIVE ARTISTS TALENT &
LITERARY AGENCY
3000 Olympic Blvd., Bldg. 4, Ste. 1200
Santa Monica, CA 90404
(310) 553-5200
T,O,Ch,F

INNOVATIVE ARTISTS YOUNG TALENT DIV.
3000 Olympic Blvd., Bldg. 4, Ste. 1200
Santa Monica, CA 90404
(310) 553-5200
Ch

INTERNATIONAL CREATIVE MGMT. (I.C.M.)
8942 Wilshire Blvd.
Beverly Hills, CA 90211
(310) 550-4000
All except Models

KAPLAN-STAHLER AGENCY
8383 Wilshire Blvd., #923
Beverly Hills, CA 90211
(310) 653-4483
T

KAZARIAN-SPENCER & ASSOC., INC.
11365 Ventura Blvd., #100
Studio City, CA 91604
(818) 769-9111
C,V,T,B,M,D,A,Ch,O,F,S,*

KERWIN AGENCY, WILLIAM
1605 N. Cahuenga, #202
Hollywood, CA 90028
 (323) 469-5155
C,T

ERIC KLASS AGENCY
139 S. Beverly Dr. #331
Beverly Hills, CA 90212
(310) 274-9169
T

KM & ASSOCIATES
4922 Vineland Avenue
N. Hollywood, CA 91601
818-766-3566

KOHNER, INC., PAUL
9300 Wilshire Blvd., #555
Beverly Hills, CA 90212
(310) 550-1060
T

L.A. TALENT, INC.
7700 W. Sunset Blvd.
Los Angeles, CA 90046
323) 656-3722
C,V,T,M,A,Ch,O,F

LANE AGENCY, STACEY
13455 Ventura Blvd., #240
Sherman Oaks, CA 91423
(818) 501-2668
C,T,Ch,V,O,D,*

LEVIN TALENT AGCY., SID
8484 Wilshire Blvd., #750
Beverly Hills, CA 90211
(323) 653-7073
C,T,Ch,F,O,*

LICHTMAN/SALNERS COMPANY
12216 Moorpark St.
Studio City, CA 91604
(818) 655-9898
T,O,F,*

LIGHT AGENCY, ROBERT
6404 Wilshire Blvd., #900
Los Angeles, CA 90048
(323) 651-1777
T,Mu,R

LINDNER & ASSOC., KEN
2049 Century Park E., #305
Los Angeles, CA 90067
(310) 277-9223
B,V

LJ & ASSOCIATES
17328 Ventura Bl. #185
Encino, CA 91316 (818) 589-6960

LOVELL & ASSOC.
6707 Milner Road
Los Angeles, CA 90068
(323) 462-1672
T,O

JANA LUKER AGENCY
1923 1/2 Westwood Blvd., #3
Los Angeles, CA 90025
(310) 441-2822
T,C,Ch,O,F,S

THE LUND AGCY, INDUSTRY
ARTISTS TALENT AGCY.
3330 Barham Blvd., South, #103
Los Angeles, CA 90068
(323) 851-6575
T,C,F,O

LYNNE & REILLY AGENCY
10725 Vanowen Street, #113
North Hollywood, CA 91605-6402
(213) 755-6434
T,C,V,R,Mu,O,Ch,S

MAJOR CLIENTS AGENCY
345 North Maple, #395
Beverly Hills, CA 90210
(310) 205-5000
C,V,T,R

MALAKY INTERNATIONAL
10642 Santa Monica Blvd., #103
Los Angeles, CA 90025
(310) 234-9114

MANN, MICHAEL TALENT
AGENCY
121 North San Vicente Blvd.
Beverly Hills, CA 90211
(323) 651-0720

MARIS AGENCY
17620 Sherman Way, #213
Van Nuys, CA 91406
(818) 708-2493
C,Mu,M

MARSHALL MODEL & TALENT
ALESE
22730 Hawthorne Bl., #201
Torrance, CA 90505
(310) 378-1223
T,C,V,A,Ch,M,O,R,B,F

MAXINE'S TALENT AGENCY
4830 Encino Ave
Encino, CA 91316
(818) 986-2946
C,T,R,S,Mu,V

MEDIA ARTISTS GROUP
6404 Wilshire Boulevard, Suite 950
Los Angeles, CA 90048 (323) 658-5050
C,T,Ch,M,O,F,B,A

MERIDIAN ARTISTS AGENCY
9229 Sunset Boulevard, #310
Los Angeles CA 90069
(310) 246-2611

METROPOLITAN TALENT AGENCY
4526 Wilshire Blvd.
Los Angeles, CA 90010
(323) 857-4500
T

MITCHELL K. STUBBS &
ASSOCIATES
1450 S. Robertson Blvd.
Los Angeles, CA 90035
310) 888-1200
C,V,T,R,B,M,Mu

MODELS GUILD OF CALIFORNIA
TALENT AGENCY
8489 W. 3rd St. #1107
Los Angeles, CA 90048
(323) 801-2132

THE MORGAN AGENCY
129 West Wilson St., #202
Costa Mesa, CA 92627
(714) 574-1120

MORRIS AGENCY, INC., WILLIAM
151 El Camino
Beverly Hills, CA 90212
(310) 274-7451
C,V,T,R,B,Mu,A,S,O,F,*

MOSS & ASSOC., H. DAVID
733 N. Seward St., P.H.
Los Angeles, CA 90038
(323) 465-1234
T,B,Ch,A,O,F,C,*

NATHE & ASSOC., SUSAN (CPC)
8281 Melrose, #200
Los Angeles, CA 90046
(323) 653-7573
C,V,O,Ch,F,*

OMNIPOP, INC.
10700 Ventura Blvd., 2nd Fl.
Studio City, CA 91604 (818) 980-9267
C,T,V,Mu,S,F,R,*

THE ORANGE GROVE GROUP,
INC.
12178 Ventura Blvd. #205
Studio City, CA 91604
(818) 762-7498
T,R,D,Mu,F,M,R,Ch,O,S,*

ORIGIN TALENT
3500 Olive Ave., 3rd Floor
Burbank, CA 9150
(818) 973-2750

OSBRINK TALENT AGENCY, CINDY
4343 Lankershim Blvd. #100
Universal City, CA 91602
(818) 760-2488
C,T,Ch,V,M

PAKULA/KING & ASSOCIATES
9229 Sunset Blvd., #315
Los Angeles, CA 90069
(310) 281-4868
T

PARADIGM, A TALENT &
LITERARY AGENCY
10100 Santa Monica Blvd., #2500
Los Angeles, CA 90067
(310) 277-4400
C,V,T,Ch,O,F,M,D

THE PARADISE GROUP
8749 Sunset Blvd., Ste. B
Los Angeles, CA 90069
(310) 854-6622

PLAYBOY MODELS
9242 Beverly Blvd.
Beverly Hills, CA 90210
(310) 246-4000
T,C,M,V,F,B

PRIVELEGE TALENT AGENCY
9229 Sunset Bl. #414
W. Hollywood, CA 90069
(310) 858-5277

PROGRESSIVE ARTISTS
400 S. Beverly, #216
Beverly Hills, CA 90212
(310) 553-8561
T

SANDERS AGENCY
8831 Sunset Blvd., #304
Los Angeles, CA 90069
(310) 652-1119
T,C,Ch,O,Mu,D,F,*

SARNOFF COMPANY, INC.
3500 West Olive Avenue, Suite 300
Burbank, CA 91505
(818) 973-4555
T,B,M

SAVAGE AGENCY, INC.
6212 Banner Ave.
Los Angeles, CA 90038
(213) 461-8316
T,C,V,Ch,R

SCAGNETTI AGENCY, JACK
5118 Vineland Ave., #102
North Hollywood, CA 91601
(818) 762-3871
C,V,T,M,O,F,D,*

SCHECHTER COMPANY, IRV
9300 Wilshire Blvd., #400
Beverly Hills, CA 90212
(310) 278-8070
T

SANDIE SCHNARR TALENT, INC.
8500 Melrose Ave., #212
W. Hollywood, Ca 90069
 (310) 360-7680
V,C

SCHOEN & ASSOC., JUDY
606 N. Larchmont Blvd., #309
Los Angeles, CA 90004
 (323) 962-1950
T

SCREEN ARTISTS AGENCY
12435 Oxnard Street
N. Hollywood, CA 91606
(818) 755-0026

SDB PARTNERS, INC.
1801 Ave. of the Stars #902
Los Angeles, CA 90067
(310) 785-0060
T

SHAPIRA & ASSOC., INC., DAVID
15821 Ventura Blvd. #235
Encino, CA 91436
(818) 906-0322
T,C,V,M

SHAPIRO-LICHTMAN STEIN
8827 Beverly Blvd.
Los Angeles, CA 90048
(310) 859-8877

SHUMAKER AGENCY
6533 Hollywood Blvd., #401
Hollywood, CA 90028
(323) 464-0745
C,R,A,Ch,Mu,O,F,S,*

SILVER, MASSETTI & SZATMARY/
WEST, Ltd.
3870 Sunset Blvd., #440
Los Angeles, CA 90069
(310) 289-0909
T,O,F

SLESSINGER & ASSOC., MICHAEL
8730 Sunset Blvd., Ste. 270
W. Hollywood, CA 90069
(310) 657-7113
T

SORICE TALENT AGCY., CAMILLE
13412 Moorpark St., #C
Sherman Oaks, CA 91423
(818) 955-1775
T,Mu,O

SPECIAL ARTISTS
345 N. Maple Dr., #302
Beverly Hills, CA 90210
310) 859-9688
C,V,M,A

SCOTT STANDER AGENCY
13701 Riverside Drive, Suite 201
Sherman Oaks, CA 91423
(818) 905-7000

STARCRAFT AGENCY
3330 Barham Boulevard, #105
Los Angeles, CA 90068
(323) 845-4784

STEVENS GROUP, THE
3518 Cahuenga Blvd., W. #306
Los Angeles, CA 90068
(323) 850-5761

STONE MANNERS
8436 West 3rd St., #740
Los Angeles, CA 90048
(323) 655-1313
T,Ch,F,O

PETER STRAIN & Assoc.
5724 W. 3rd Street, # 302
Los Angeles, CA 90036
(323) 525-3391

THE SUN AGENCY
8961 Sunset Blvd., Ste. D
Los Angeles, CA 90069
(310) 888-8737
C,V,T,R,M,D,B,Ch,Mu,O,F,S

SUTTON-BARTH-VENNARI, INC.
145 S. Fairfax Ave., #310
Los Angeles, CA 90036
(323) 938-6000
C,V

SWB THEATRICAL
8383 Wilshire Blvd., 850
Beverly Hills, CA 90211
(323) 655-0069

TALENT GROUP, INC.
6300 Wilshire Blvd., #900
Los Angeles, CA 90048
(323) 852-9559
T,C,V,M,F,Ch,R,B

THE TALENT SYNDICATE, LLC
1680 N. Vine Street, Suite 614
Los Angeles, CA 90028
(323) 463-7300
C,V,Mu,O,F,*

TANNEN & ASSOC., HERB
10801 National Blvd. #101
Los Angeles, CA 90064
(310) 466-5822
C,V,T,Ch,O,F

THOMAS TALENT AGENCY
6709 LaTijera, #915
Los Angeles, CA 90045
(310) 665-0000
T,D,C,Mu,F

THORNTON & ASSOC., ARLENE
12001 Ventura Blvd., #201
Studio City, CA 91604-2609
 (818) 760-6688
C,V,R,B

TISHERMAN AGENCY
6767 Forest Lawn Dr., #101
Los Angeles, CA 90068
(323) 850-6767
C,V,OB,F,*

A TOTAL ACTING EXPERIENCE
5353 Topanga Canyon Road, Suite 220
Woodland Hills, CA 91364
 (818) 340-9249 ALL AREAS

TURTLE AGENCY
955 S. Carillo Dr. #200
Los Angeles, CA 90048
(323) 954-4066
T

TWO ANGELS AGENCY
2026 Cliff Drive, Suite 200
Santa Barbara, A 93109
 (805) 957-9654

UNITED ARTISTS TALENT
AGENCY
14011 Ventura Blvd. #213
Sherman Oaks. CA 91423
(818) 788-7305

UNITED TALENT AGENCY
9560 Wilshire Boulevard
Beverly Hills, CA 90212
(310)-273-6700

THE VISSION AGENCY
1801 Century Park E., 24th floor
Los Angeles, CA 90067
(310) 553-8833

THE WALLIS AGENCY
4444 Riverside Drive, #105
Burbank, CA 91505
(818) 953-4848
T,C,V,O,F

WARDLOW & ASSOC. (Formerly
Camden)
1501 Main Street, #204
Venice, CA 90291
(310) 452-1292
T

WATERS & NICOLOSI
9301 Wilshire Blvd., #300
Beverly Hills, CA 90210
(310) 777-8277

WAUGH AGENCY, ANN
4741 Laurel Canyon Blvd., Ste 200
North Hollywood, CA 91607
(818) 980-0141
T,V,C,Ch,O,F,*

WEIGLE, JUDITH TALENT
AGENCY
6505 Green Valley Circle, #203
Culver City, CA 90230
310-641-9109

WILSON & ASSOC., SHIRLEY
5410 Wilshire Blvd., # 806
Los Angeles, CA 90036
(323) 857-6977
C,T,Ch,F,O

WRITERS & ARTISTS AGENCY
8383 Wilshire Blvd., #550
Los Angeles, CA 90211
(323) 866-0900
T,Ch,O,F

ZADEH & ASSOC., STELLA
5435 Balboa Blvd., #212
Encino, CA 91316
818-501-0800
B,T

ZANUCK, PASSON & PACE, INC.
13317 Ventura Blvd., Ste. I
Sherman Oaks, CA 91423
(818) 783-4890

MIAMI AGENTS

ALLIANCE TALENT
1940 Harrison Street, #300
Hollywood, FL 33020
(954) 927-0072

AZUREE MODELING & TALENT
AGCY
140 N. Orlando Ave., #120
Winter Park, FL 32789
(407) 629-5025
M,C,V,If,Ch,O,F,*,S,T,NB,Id,P

BERG TALENT AGNECY
15908 Eagle River Way
Tampa FL 33624
(813) 877-5533
M,D,B,A,Ch,O,F,C,V,If,T,CD,In,Id,P

BOCA TALENT & MODEL
AGENCY
829 SE 9th Street Palm Plaza Suite 4
Deerfield Beach, FL 33441
(305) 428-4677

851 North Market Street
Jacksonville, FL 32202
f(904) 354-5753
C,V,T,B,M,D,A,CH,O,F,*,S

BREVARD TALENT GROUP
405 Palm Springs Blvd.
Indian Harbor Beach, FL 32937
(407) 773-1355
Ch,O,F,C,If,T,CD,In,NB,Id,P

CENTRAL FLORIDA CASTING, INC.
2601 Wells Avenue, Suite 181
Fern Park, FL 32730
(407) 830-9226

COCONUT GROVE TALENT
3525 Vista Court
Miami, FL 33133
(305) 858-3002

DIMENSIONS III MODEL & TALENT
5205 S. Orange Ave., #209
Orlando, FL 32809
(407) 851-2575
M,D,Ch,O,F,*,C,V,If,T,CD,It,NB,Id,P

THE DIAMOND AGENCY
204 West Bay Avenue
Longwood, FL 32750
(407) 830-4040

GREEN & GREEN MODEL &
TALENT AGCY.
1688 Meridian Ave., #1000
Miami Beach, FL 33139
(305) 532-9880
M,Ch,O,F,*,C,V,R,If,T,CD,IN,NB,Id,P

HURT-GARVER TALENT
400 N. New York Ave., #207
Winter Park, FL 32789-3159
(407) 740-5700
M,D,C,V,If,Ch,O,F,T,CD,In,NB,Id,P

KOLDENHOVEN & ASSOCIATES
d.b.a The Christensen Group
235 Coastline Road
Sanford, FL 32771
407) 302-2272

MARIE INC., IRENE
728 Ocean Dr.
Miami Beach, FL 33139-6203
Dade (305) 672-2344
Broward (954) 771-1400
M,A,Ch,O,F,*,C,R,If,T,CD,In,NB,Id,P

MARTIN - DONALDS INC., DBA
1915A Hollwood Blvd.
Hollywood, FL 33020
(954) 921-2321
All Areas

ROXANNE McMILLAN TALENT
AGCY
12100 N.E. 16th Ave., #106
N. Miami, FL 33161
(305) 899-9150
ALL AREAS - No News/Broadcast/Rec.

POLAN TALENT AGENCY,
MARION
10 N.E. 11th Ave.
Ft. Lauderdale, Fl 33301
(954) 525-8351
M,D,B,A,Mu,C,If,Ch,O,F,*,S,T,CD,It,NB,Id,P

Agent Specializing in Spanish
language

POMMIER MODELS, MICHELE
81 Washington Ave.
Miami Beach, FL 33139
(305) 672-9344
ALL AREAS - No *

SHEFFIELD AGENCY,
P.O. Box 101418 (mailing address only)
Fort Lauderdale, FLA 33310
 (954) 523-5887
(Please call AFTRA for agency office location)

STELLAR TALENT AGENCY
407 Lincoln Rd., Ste. 2K
Miami Beach, FL 33139 (305) 672-2217
CH,D,F,M,O,*,C,T,V

STRICKLY SPEAKING,
711 Executive Dr.
Winter Park, FL 32789 (407) 645-2111
V,If,F,CD,In,NB,Id,P

WORLD OF KIDS, INC.
1460 Ocean Drive, #205
Miami Beach, FL 33139 (305) 672-5437
C,V,T,M,D,Mu,Ch,*

NASHVILLE AGENTS

AGENCY FOR THE PERFORMING ARTS
3322 West End Ave., Suite 520
Nashville, TN 31203
(615) 297-0100

CREATIVE ARTISTS AGENCY
3310 West End Ave., 5th Fl.
Nashville, TN 37203
(615) 383-8787

DS ENTERTAINMENT
30 Music Square West, Suite 158
Nashville, TN 37203
 (615) 782-0211

LEE ATTRACTIONS INC.,(TN), BUDDY
38 Music Square E., #300
Nashville, TN 37203
(615) 244-4336

MORRIS AGENCY INC., WILLIAM
2100 West End Ave., Suite 1000
P.O. Box 37203
Nashville, TN 37203
(615) 385-0310

TALENT & MODEL LAND INC.
P.O. Box 40763
Nashville, TN 37204
(615) 321-5596

TALENT TREK
2021 21st Avenue, South, Suite 102
Nashville, TN 37212
(615) 279-0010

TALENT TREK AGENCY
1701 West End Ave., #100
Nashville, TN 37203-2601
 (615) 244-6411

NEW YORK AGENTS

ABOUT ARTISTS AGENCY
355 Lexington Avenue
New York, NY 10017 (212) 490-7191
Mu,V,R,If,T,CD,NB,Id,P

ABRAMS ARTISTS & ASSOC.
275 Seventh Avenue
26th Floor
New York, NY 10001
646-486-4600
All Areas

ACCESS TALENT, INC.
37 East 28th St., Suite 500
New York, NY 10016 (212) 684-7795
VOICE   OVER:
B,O,F,C,R,If,T,It,NB,Id,P

ACME TALENT & LITERARY
875 Avenue of the Americas, Suite 2108
New York, NY 10001
 (212) 328-0388
C,V,T,Mu,Ch,O,F,*

ACTUAL TALENT
1260 New Britain Rd # 65
West Hartford, CT 06110
Phone: (860) 920-5322
Fax: (860) 561-2473
Ch, C, F, If, CD, P, Id, O, R, T, V, NB, M

ATLAS TALENT AGENCY, INC.
36 West 44th Street, Suite 1000
York, NY 10036
212-730-4500

BRET ADAMS LTD.
448 44th St.
New York, NY 10036
(212) 765-5630
D,Mu,O,R,T,In

AGENCY FOR THE PERFORMING
ARTS
888 Seventh Ave.
New York, NY 10106
(212) 582-1500
Mu,O,F,S,T

AGENTS FOR THE ARTS, INC.
203 West 23rd St., 3rd Fl.
New York, NY 10011
(212) 229-2562
D,B,Mu,C,V,O,*,T,NB,Id,P

ALLIANCE TALENT, inc.
1501 Broadway, #404
New York, NY 10036
(212) 840-6868 D,Mu,T,CD,It

AMATO AGENCY, MICHAEL
1650 Broadway, RM #307
New York, NY 10019
(212) 247-4456
A,B,Ch,C,M,O,F,If,T,In

AMERICAN INT'L TALENT
AGENCY
303 West 42nd St., #608
New York, NY 10036
(212) 245-8888
C,Ch,D,F,Id,If,M,Mu,NB,O,*,P,R,S,T,V

ANDERSON, BEVERLY
1501 Broadway, #2008
New York, NY 10036 (212) 944-7773
D,Mu,O,F,V,C,R,T,In

ANDREADIS TALENT AGENCY
119 West 57th St., #711
New York, NY 10019
(212) 315-0303
All Areas

ARTIST'S AGENCY INC.
230 W. 55th St.
New York, NY 10019
(212) 245-6960

THE ARTISTS GROUP EAST
1650 Broadway, Suite 711
New York, NY 10019 (212) 586-1452
Mu, O,F,T,Id

ASSOCIATED BOOKING CORP.
1995 Broadway, #501
New York, NY 10023
 (212) 874-2400
Mu,C,R,T,CD,It,Id

ASTOR AGENCY, THE, RICHARD
250 West 57th St., #2014
New York, NY 10107
(212) 581-1970
D,Mu,O,F,T

BARRY HAFT BROWN ARTISTS
AGENCY
165 West 46th St., #908
New York, NY 10036
(212) 869-9310
D,C,T

BAUMAN REDANTY & SHAUL
250 West 57th St., #473
New York, NY 10019
(212) 757-0098
A,B,D,F,M,MU,O,S,*,R,T,V

BEILIN AGENCY INC., PETER
230 Park Ave., RM #923
New York, NY 10169
(212) 949-9119
ALL AREAS - EXCEPT CHILDREN

BERMAN, BOALS & FLYNN, INC.
230 West 30th Street, Suite 401
New York, NY 10001
212-868-1068

BIENSTOCK INC., N.S.
1740 Broadway, 24th Fl.
New York, NY 10019
(212) 765-3040
Mu,C,V,B,R,If,Ch,O,F,*,S,T,CD,In,NB,Id,P

BUCHWALD & ASSOC., DON
10 East 44th St.
New York, NY 10017
(212) 867-1200
M,D,B,Ch,O,F,*,S,C,V,R,If,T,CD,It,NB,Id,P

CARLSON-MENASHE ARTISTS
149 5th Avenue, #1204
New York, NY 10010
212-228-8826
C,V,T,Id

CARRY COMPANY
49 West 46th Street, 4th Floor
New York, NY 10036
(212) 768-2793

CARSON-ADLER AGENCY, INC.
250 West 57th St.
New York, NY 10107
(212) 307-1882
CH,C

CARSON ORGANIZATION, LTD.,
240 West 44th St., PH
New York, NY 10036
(212) 221-1517
C,V,R,Ch,T

COLEMAN-ROSENBERG
155 East 55th St., 5D
New York, NY 10022
(212) 838-0734
F,O,T

COLUMBIA ARTISTS
MANAGEMENT
165 West 57th Street
New York, NY 10019
(212) 397-6900

CORNERSTONE TALENT AGENCY
132 West 22nd St., fl 4
New York, NY 10011
 (212) 807-8344
D,C,V,R,O,F,*,S,T,Id

CUNNINGHAM, ESCOTT, DIPENE
& ASSOC.
257 Park Avenue South, Suite 900
New York, NY 10010
(212) 477-1666
ALL AREAS

DICCE TALENT AGENCY, GINGER
56 W. 45th St. #1100
New York, NY 10036
(212) 974-7455
M,C,VO,If,Ch,O,F,S,T,CD,NB,Id,P

DOUGLAS, GORMAN,
ROTHACKER & WILHELM, INC.
1501 Broadway, #703
New York, NY 10036
(212) 382-2000
Mu,R,O,F,If,T,Id

DUVA – FLACK, assoc.
200 West 57th St., #1008
New York, NY 10019
(212) 957-9600
D,Mu,O,F,T,CD,In

DULCINA EISEN ASSOCIATES
154 East 61st St.
New York, NY 10021
(212) 355-6617
D,Mu,O,F,*,C,R,T,Id

EWCR & ASSOCIATES
311 West 43rd St., #304
New York, NY 10036
(212) 586-9110
Ch, T, ACTORS

FAMOUS ARTISTS AGENCY INC.
1700 Broadway
New York, NY 10019
(212) 245-3939

FLAUNT MODEL MANAGEMENT
114 East 32nd Street
New York, NY 10016
(212) 679-9011
M,C,V,If,O,F,T,CD,In,NB,Id,P

FRESH FACES AGENCY, INC.
108 South Franklin Avenue, Suite 11
Valley Stream, NY 11580
 (516) 223-0034
M,D,Mu,Ch,O in all areas

FRONTEIR BOOKING INT'L, INC.
1560 Broadway, #1110
New York, NY 10036
(212) 221-0220
M,C,V,Ch,F,T,CD,Id

GAGE GROUP, THE
315 West 57th St., #4H
New York, NY 10019
(212) 541-5250
C,V,B,R,In,T,CD,In,NB,Id,P

GARBER TALENT AGENCY
2 Penn Plaza
New York, NY 10121-0099
(212) 292-4910
C,V,T,R,D,Mu,O,F,*

GENERATION TV
20 West 20th Street, #1008
New York NY 10011
(646) 230-9491

THE GERSH AGENCY NY INC., THE
130 West 42nd St., #2400
New York, NY 10036
(212) 997-1818
T

THE GILCHRIST TALENT GROUP, INC.,
630 Ninth Ave., Ste 800
New York, NY 10036
(212) 2203532/33
D,Mu,Ch,O,C,V,T,Id

HADLEY ENTERPRISES LTD., PEGGY
250 West 57th St.
New York, NY 10107
(212) 246-2166
D,Mu,R,F,T

HARDEN-CURTIS ASSOCIATES
850 Seventh Ave., #405
New York, NY 10019
(212) 977-8502
O,F,* ,T,Id

HARTIG AGENCY,, LTD., MICHAEL
156 Fifth Ave., Suite 820
New York, NY 10010
(212) 929-1772
D,Mu,O,S,C,V,R,If,T,In,P

HENDERSON/HOGAN AGENCY, INC.
850 Seventh Ave., #1003
New York, NY 10019
(212) 765-5190
D,Mu,C,V,R,If,Ch,O,*,T,Id,P

THE BARBARA HOGENSON AGENCY
165 West End Avenue, Suite 19-C
New York, NY 10023
(212) 874-8084
V,R,T,CD,In

HWA TALENT REPRESENTATIVES
220 East 23rd St., #400
New York, NY 10010
(212) 889-0800
M,D,Mu,C,V,R,If,O,F,T,CD,It,NB,Id,P

INGBER & ASSOCIATES
274 Madison Ave., #1104
New York, NY 10016
(212) 889-9450
O,F,C,V,R,If,CD,In,NB,Id,P

INNOVATIVE ARTISTS TALENT & LITERARY AGENCY
141 5th Avenue, 3rd Fl. South
New York, NY 10010
(212) 253-6900
T - Ch,O,F

INTERNATIONAL CREATIVE
MGMT. (I.C.M)
40 West 57th St.
New York, NY 10019
212) 556-5600
All except Models

JAN J. AGENCY, INC.
365 West 34th Street, Fl #2
New York, NY 10001
(212) 967-5265
C,V,R,If,Ch,F,*,T,CD,In,Id,P

JORDAN, GILL & DORNBAUM
AGCY
156 Fifth Ave., #711
New York, NY 10010
(212) 463-8455
M,D,C,V,Ch,F,T,CD,In,NB,Id,P

KAHN, INC., JERRY
853 Seventh Ave.
New York, NY 10019
(212) 245-7317
D,F,MU,O,C,R,T,V

KERIN-GOLDBERG ASSOCIATES
155 East 55th St., #5D
New York, NY 10022
(212) 838-7373
D,Mu,Ch,O,F,*,S,If,In,B,T,CD,It

KING, LTD., ARCHER
317 West 46th Street, Suite 3A
New York, NY 10035
(212) 765-3103

KOLSTEIN TALENT AGENCY dba
NAOMI'S WORLD OF
ENTERTAINMENT, INC.
85 C Lafayette Avenue
Suffern, NY 10901
845) 357-8301
All Areas

KRASNY OFFICE, INC.,
1501 Broadway, #1303
New York, NY 10036
 (212) 730-8160
D,A,Mu,C,V,If,O,F,T,CD,NB,Id,P

L.B.H. ASSOC., INC.
20 West 64th St., Apt.302
New York, NY 10023
(212) 501-8936

BIG BANDS, JAZZ
LALLY TALENT AGENCY
630 Ninth Ave., #800
New York, NY 10036
(212) 974-8718
D,Mu,R,O,F,*,T

LANTZ OFFICE, THE
200 West 57th St., # 503
New York, NY 10019
(212) 586-0200

LARNER, LTD., LIONEL
119 West 57th St., #1412
New York, Ny 10019
(212) 246-3105
C,TV

BERNARD LIEBHABER AGENCY
352 Seventh Ave., fl 7
New York, NY 10001
(212)-631-7561
V,T,Ch,O,F

THE LEUDTKE AGENCY
1674 Broadway, Ste. 7A
New York, NY 10019
(212) 220-3532
All areas - except models

LEVY AGENCY, BRUCE
311 West 43rd St., #602
New York, NY 10036,
(212) 262-6845
A,B,D,F,M,MU,O,S,*,C,R,T,V

MCCULLOUGH Assoc.
8 S. Hanover Ave.
Margate, NJ 08402
(609) 822-2222
M,C,If,F,T,Id,P

MEREDITH MODEL MGMT.
10 Furler St.
Totawa, NJ 07512
(651) 812-0122
M,Ch,O,F,*,C,V,NB,Id

JMA - THE JACK MENASHE
AGENCY
160 East 61st Street, 3rd Fl.
New York, NY 10021
(212) 588-0902/0903
TV Prog - D,Mu,O,F,NB,Id

MORRIS AGENCY, WILLIAM
1325 Ave. of The Americas
New York, NY 10019
(212) 586-5100
A,B,D,F,M,MU,O,S,*,C,R,T,V

NOUVELLE TALENT INC.
453 West 17th St., #3
New York, NY 10011
(212) 645- 0940
M,F,Id,P

OMNIPOP INC., TALENT AGENCY
55 West Old Country Rd.
Hicksville, NY 11801
(516) 937-6011
C,V,B,R,If,T,CD,NB,Id,P

OPPENHEIM-CHRISTIE ASSOC.,
LTD.
13 East 37th St.
New York, NY 10016
(212) 213-4330
F,C,V,If,CD,In,NB,Id,P

OSCARD AGENCY, INC., FIFI
24 West 40th St., 17th Fl.
New York, NY 10018
(212) 764-1100
M,C,V,If,Ch,T,CD,It,NB,Id,P

PARADIGM
200 West 57th St., #900
New York, NY 10019
(212) 246-1030
C,V,T,If,P,Id,M,D,Ch,O,F

PROFESSIONAL ARTISTS
UNLIMITED
321 West 44th Street, #605
New York, NY 10036
(212) 247-8770
D,B,Mu,R,If,O,F,T

PYRAMID ENTERTAINMENT
89 Fifth Avenue.
New York, NY 10003
(212) 242-7274

RADIOACTIVE TALENT INC.
350 Third Avenue, Suite 400
New York, NY 10010

REICH AGENCY, INC., NORMAN
1650 Broadway, Suite 303
New York, NY 10019
(212) 399-2881
B,A,C,V,Id

ROOS LTD., GILLA
16 West 22nd St., 7th Fl.
New York, NY 10010
(212) 727-7820

SAMES & ROLLNICK ASSOC.
250 West 57th St., RM #703
New York, NY 10107
(212) 315-4434
D,Mu,O,F,T

SANDERS AGENCY LTD., THE
1204 Broadway, #306
New York, NY 10001
(212) 779-3737

SCHIFFMAN, EKMAN,
MORRISON & MARX,inc
(S.E.M & M)
22 West 19th St., 8th Fl.
New York, NY 10011
(212) 627-5500
M,D,B,A,Mu,Ch,O,F,*,S,C,V,R,If,T,CD,In,NB,Id,P

SCHILL AGENCY, INC., WILLIAM
302A West 12th Street, #183
New York, NY 10014
(877) 813-3923
D,Mu,Ch,O,F,*,C,T,Id,P

SCHULLER TALENT / NEW YORK
KIDS
276 Fifth Ave.
New York, NY 10001
 (212) 532-6005

SILVER, MASSETTI & SZATMARY/
EAST LTD.
145 West 45th St., #1204
New York, NY 10036
(212) 391-4545
TV PROGRAMS ONLY

ANN STEELE AGENCY
240 West 44th Street, #1
Helen Hayes Theatre
New York, NY 10036
(212) 278-0896
Actors:D,Mu,Ch,O,F,C,V,T,CD,NB,Id,P

STRAIN & ASSOC., INC., PETER
1501 Broadway, #2900
New York, NY 10036
(212) 391-0380

TALENT REPRESENTATIVE, INC.
20 East 53rd St.
New York, NY 10022
 (212) 752-1835
C,V,R,If,T,Id

TAMAR WOLBROM, INC.
130 West 42nd Street, #707
New York, NY 10036
(212) 398-4595
B,C,VO,R,If,T,CD,NB,Id,P

THE TANTLEFF OFFICE
375 Greenwich St., #603
New York, NY 10013
(212) 941-3939
D,Mu,R,F,T,Id,P

TRANUM, ROBERTSON &
HUGHES
600 Madison Avenue
New York, NY 10017
(212) 371-7500
M,C,V,R,If,Ch,CD,Id,P

UNIVERSAL ATTRACTIONS INC.
225 West 57th Street
New York, NY 10019
(212) 582-7575
Mu

WATERS & NICOLOSI
1501 Broadway, #1305
New York, NY 10036
(212) 302-8787
Ch,O,F,T

WRIGHT REPRESENTATIVES, ANN
165 West 46th St., #1105
New York, NY 10036
(212) 764-6770
M,D,B,A,Mu,C,V,O,F,*,Id,P

WRITERS & ARTISTS AGENCY
19 West 44th St., #1000
New York, NY 10036
(212) 391-1112
Ch,O,F,S,C,V,R,If,T,It

PHILADELPHIA AGENTS

ASKINS MODELS, DENISE
55 North Third Street
Philadelphia, PA 19106
(215) 925-7795
M,C,V,If,Ch,O,F,T,NB,Id,P

CLARO AGENCY INC., 1
513 W. Passyunk Ave.
Philadelphia, PA 19145
 (215) 465-7788
M,D,B,Ch,O,F,C,V,R,If,T,CD,It,NB,Id,P

EXPRESSIONS MODELING & TALENT
110 Church St.
Philadelphia, PA 19106
(215) 923-4420
M,D,C,V,If,Ch,O,F,*,T,NB,Id,P

GOODMAN AGENCY
605 West Rt. 70
Cherry Hill, NJ 08002
(609) 795-7979 (actors)
(609) 795-3133 (clients)

GREER LANGE ASSOC.
40 Lloyd Ave., #104
Malvern, PA 19355
(610) 647-5515
M,C,V,If,O,F,*,CD,In,NB,Id,P

MCCULLOUGH ASSOC.
8 S. Hanover Avenue Atlantic City,
NJ 08402-2615
(609) 822-2222
M,D,A,O,F,C,If,T,Id,P

MODELS ON THE MOVE
1200 Route 70, Ste. 6
Barclay Towers
P.O. Box 4037
Cherry Hills, NJ 08034
(609) 667-1060
M,D,B,A,Mu,Ch,O,F,*,S,C,V,If,T,Id,P

PLAZA 7
160 North Gulph Road
King of Prussia, PA 19406
(610) 337-2693
M,C,V,If,Ch,O,F,*,S,T,NB,Id,P

REINHARD AGENCY
2021 Arch St., Suite 404
Philadelphia, PA 19103
(215) 567-2008
All Areas - No Musical Artists

PHOENIX AGENTS

ACTION TALENT
2720 East Broadway Boulevard
Tucson, AZ 85716
520-881-6535
M,B,Mu,Ch,O,F,*,S,C,V,R,If,T,CD,It,NB,Id,P

FORD/BLACK AGENCY, ROBERT
4300 N Miller road, #202
Scottsdale, AZ 85251
(480) 966-2537
(480) 967-5424 (fax)

M,B,A,C,V,If,Ch,O,F,*,S,TCD,It,NB,Id,P
DANI'S AGENCY
1 E. Camelback Rd., #550
Phoenix, AZ 85012
(602) 263-1918
ALL AREAS - No News,*,Variety

FOSIS MODELING & TALENT
AGENCY
2777 N. Campbell Ave., #209
Tucson, AZ 85719
(520) 795-3534

LEIGHTON AGENCY
2375 East Camelback, fl 5
Phoenix, AZ 85016
(602) 224-9255
M,C,V,R,If,Ch,O,F,T,CD,It,NB,Id,P

SIGNATURE MODELS & TALENT
AGENCY
2600 N. 44th Street, Ste.#209
Phoenix, AZ 85008
(602) 966-1102
ALL AREAS - No Musical Artists

PITTSBURGH AGENTS

THE TALENT GROUP
2820 Smallman St.
Pittsburgh, PA 15222
(412) 471-8011
M,B,C,V,If,Ch,O,F,*,T,CD,It,NB,Id,P

DOCHERTY, INC.
109 Market Street
Pittsburgh, PA 15222
412-765-1400
ALL AREAS

PORTLAND AGENTS

CUSICK'S TALENT MGMT.
1009 N.W. Hoyt, #100
Portland, OR 97209
(503) 274-8555
ALL EXCEPT *

ERHART TALENT
037 SW Hamilton Street
Portland, OR 97201
(503) 243-6362
M,B,C,V,N,R,If,Ch,O,F,*,S,T,CD,It,NB,Id

MASHIA TALENT MANAGEMENT
2808 NE Martin Luther King, Jr. Boulevard, #L
Portland, OR 97212
(503) 331-9293
C,V,SR,If,T,In,N,Id

ROSE CITY TALENT
239 NW 13th Ave., Ste 215
Portland, OR 97209
(503) 274-1005

WILSON Entertain.
See Erhart Talent

RACINE-KENOSHA AGENTS

LINS LTD. LORI
7611 West Holmes
Greenfield, WI 53220
(414) 282-3500

WILSON TALENT (WI), ARLENE
809 S. 60th St., Suite 201
Milwaukee, WI 53214
 (414) 223-0100

SAN DIEGO AGENTS

AGENCY 2 MODEL & TALENT (SD)
1717 Kettner Blvd., #200
San Diego, CA 92101
(619) 645-7744

ARTIST MGMT.inc
835 Fifth Ave., #411
San Diego, CA 92101
(619) 233-6655

ELEGANCE MODEL & TALENT
2763 State Street
Carlsbad, CA 92008
(619) 434-3397

JET SET TALENT
AGENCY
2160 Avenida de la Playa
La Jolla, CA 92037
(858) 551-9393
C,NB,SR,IF,T,IT

NOUVEAU MODEL & TALENT
909 Prospect Street, #230
San Diego, CA 92037
(619) 456-1400

SAN DIEGO MODEL
MGMT.
438 Camino Del Rio N., #116
San Diego, CA 92108
(619) 296-1018
CH, D, M, O, C, V

SHAMON FREITAS & co
9606 Tierra Grande St., #204
San Diego, CA 92126
(619) 234-3043

SAN FRANCISCO AGENTS

AFFINITY MODELS & TALENT
873-B Sutter Street
San Francisco, CA 94109
415-409-9991

BOOM MODELS & TALENT AGCY.
2325 Third Street, #223
San Francisco, CA 94107
(415) 626-6591
M,A,C,V,R,If,Ch,O,F,*,S,T,CD,It,NB,Id,P

FILM-THEATRE ACTORS
EXCHANGE
3145 Geary Blvd., # 752
San Francisco, CA 94118
(415) 379-9308
C,V,T,CD,It,NB,Id

GENERATIONS MODEL & TALENT
AGENCY
340 Brannan Street, #302
San Francisco, CA 94107
(415) 777-9099
C,V,T,M,Ch,O,F,*,S

J.E. TALENT, LLC
323 Geary Street, #302
San Francisco, CA 94102
(415) 395-9475
C,V,R,If,T,In,NB,Id,P

LOOK MODEL & TALENT
166 Geary Blvd., #1406
San Francisco, CA 94108
(415) 781-2841
M,B,Mu,C,V,If,Ch,O,F,*,T,CD,It,NB,Id,P

MARLA DELL TALENT
2124 Union Street
San Francisco, CA 94123
(415) 563-9213
M,A,C,V,R,Ch,O,F,T,CD,It,NB,Id,P

PANDA TALENT AGENCY
3721 Hoen Ave.
Santa Rosa, CA 95405
(707) 576-0711
M,D,A,Mu,C,V,Ch,O,F,*,S,T,CD,NB,Id,P

STARS-THE AGENCY (SF)
23 Grant Avenue, 4th Floor
San Francisco, CA 94108
(415) 421-6272
ALL AREAS

TALENT PLUS AGENCY/LOS
LATINOS
(HISPANIC DIVISION)

DYER BUILDING
2801 Moorpark Ave., #11
San Jose, CA 95128
(408) 296-2213
ALL AREAS - No *

TONRY TALENT
885 Bryant Street, Ste. 201
San Francisco, CA 94103
(415) 543-3797
M,Ch,O,F,*,C,V,B,If,T,It,NB,Id,P

TOP MODELS & TALENT AGENCY
The Flood Building
870 Market St., Suite 1076
San Francisco, CA 94102
 (415) 391-1800
M,B,Mu,C,V,If,Ch,O,F,*,S,CD,It,NB,Id,P

SEATTLE AGENTS

ACTORS GROUP (WA), THE
114 Alaskan Way, S. #104
Seattle, WA 98104
(206) 624-9465

COLLEEN BELL MODELING &
TALENT AGENCY
14205 SE 36th St, #100
Bellevue, WA 98006
(425) 649-1111

DRAMATIC ARTISTS AGENCY
1000 Lenora Street, #511
Seattle, WA 98121
(206) 442-9190

ENTCO INTERNATIONAL, Inc.
7017 196TH ST SW
Lynnwood, WA 98036
(425) 670-0777

HEFFNER MANAGEMENT
Westlake Center
1601 Fifth Ave., Suite 2301
Seattle, WA 98101
(206) 622-2211

KID BIZ TALENT
One Bellevue Center
411 108th Ave.,N.E.,#2050
Bellevue, WA 98004
 (425) 455-8800

SEATTLE MODELS GUILD
1809 Seventh Ave., Suite 303
Seattle, WA 98101
(206) 622-1406

TOPO SWOPE TALENT AGENCY
1932 1st Ave., Suite 700
Seattle, WA 98101
(206) 443-2021

ST. LOUIS AGENTS

CITY TALENT
2101 Locust Street, Suite 2 West
St. Louis MO 63103
(314) 621-7200
M,CI,V,If,Ch,O,F,*,TV,CD,It,NB,Id,P

PRIMA MODELS
522 A. S. Henley Rd.
St. Louis, MO 63105
(314) 721-1235
CH,D,F,M,O,*,C,T,V

THE QUINN AGENCY
1062 Madison Street
St. Charles, MO 63301
(636) 947-0120
Mu,R,Ch,F,*,S,NB

TALENT PLUS INC. (ST. LOUIS)
1222 Lucas, Suite 300
St. Louis, MO 63103
(314) 421-9400
M,C,V,R,If,Ch,O,F,*,S,CD,It,NB,Id,P

TRI-STATE AGENTS

ACT 1 AGENCY
6100 N. Keystone
Indianapolis, Indiana 46220
(317) 255-3100
M,C,V,If,Ch,O,F,NB,Id,P

CAM TALENT-CINCINATTI
1150 W. Eight St., #262
Cincinnati, OH 45203
(513) 421-1795
M,B,C,V,If,Ch,O,F,*,T,CD,NB,Id,P

CREATIVE TALENT
5864 Nike Dr.
Hilliard, OH 43026
(614) 294-7827
M,D,B,A,Mu,Ch,O,F,*,S

GOENNER TALENT, JO
10019 Paragon Rd.
Dayton, OH 45458
(937) 885—2595
M,D,B,C,V,If,Ch,O,F,*,S,T,NB,Id,P

GOENNER TALENT, JO
3141 Exon Avenue
Cincinnati, OH 45241
(513) 733-3330

HEYMAN TALENT, INC
3308 Brotherton
Cincinnati, OH 45209
(513) 533-3113
M,B,C,V,B,If,Ch,O,F,*,T,NB,It,NB,Id

HELEN WELLS Agency
401 Pennsylvania Pkwy.
Indianapolis, IN 46280
(317) 843-5363
C,V,M,Ch,O,F,*

TWIN CITIES AGENTS

CARYN MODEL & TALENT
Butler Square Bldg.
100 N. 6th St., #270B
Minneapolis, MN 55403
(612) 349-3600
M,B,A,C,V,R,If,Ch,O,F,*,T,CD,NB,Id,P

JOE KATZ MODELS
701 - 4th Ave South, #1700
Minneapolis, MN 55415
(612) 377-7630
C,T,R,B

MEREDITH MODEL & TALENT
800 Washington Avenue North,
Suite 511
Minneapolis, MN 55401
(612) 340-9555
ALL AREAS

MOORE CREATIVE TALENT, INC.
(Formally Eleanor Moore Agency
and Creative Casting)
1610-B West Lake Street
Minneapolis, MN 55408
(612) 827-3823
M,D,A,C,If,Ch,O,F,*,T,In,CD,NB,Id,P

NEW FACES MODELS & TALENT
INC.
6301 Wayzata Blvd.
Minneapolis, MN 55416
(612) 544-8668
M,D,A,C,V,R,If,Ch,O,F,*,S,T,CD,NB,Id,P

THE WEHMANN AGENCY
1128 Harmon Place, #205
Minneapolis, MN 55403
(612) 333-6393
M,B,A,C,V,If,Ch,O,F,*,S,CD,NB,Id

WASHINGTON AGENTS

THE BULLOCK AGENCY
5200 Bullock Avenue, #102
Hyattsville, MD 20781
(301) 905-9598
All Areas - except Athletes

KIDS INTERNATIONAL
938 East Swan Creek Rd., Suite 152
Ft. Washington, MD 20744
(301) 292-6094

TAYLOR-ROYALL, Inc.
6247 Falls Road
Baltimore, MD 21209
(410) 466-5000
C,R,T,V

For updated current lists of franchised talent agencies in your area, contact the Screen Actor's Guild or AFTRA office nearest you.

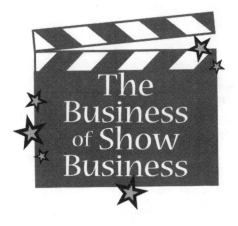

Chapter 8

Managers

**"Do not tell others what they ought to do,
but you do as you ought."**

Epictetus

Do you need a manager? That depends on who you are and how successful your career is. Times are changing at a significant rate. Many artists think they will succeed more quickly by hiring a manager as well as an agent. Here are a few things to keep in mind. Although it appears that both agents and managers serve similar functions, there are distinctions between them. A manager is supposed to direct your career, give advice, introduce talent to casting people and "manage" an actors business. An agent negotiates contracts and books talent on jobs. Actors and managers can work together. Whereas talent agencies are required to be licensed in many states, managers are not, therefore you need to be cautious in contracting for the services of a manager. Managers charge anywhere from 10% to 25% of your gross. This percentage is in addition to any agency fees. Many management contracts stipulate that all extensions, renewals, or renegotiations of employment contracts are commissionable, even after the expiration of the management contract. This means that even if you have terminated your manager, that manager may be entitled to commissions on any jobs with the same employer. There are also clauses which contend that if you get fired, the manager still will receive a commission on what you would have been paid if you were not terminated. It is imperative that you carefully read, and have your attorney read, any contract before signing it. Sign only for a brief period, one or two years to make sure this manager is right for you.

Managers are not franchised or regulated by SAG and AFTRA. Although the unions may be able to answer questions for you, they will not be able to arbitrate or resolve disputes between a manager and talent, even if the talent is union. There are well established firms in the business of personal management and business management. Again, most of these firms handle big name clients and do not advertise or solicit for talent. For more information on managers, call the Conference of Personal Managers at 310-275-2456.

Most management contracts stipulate that all work is commissionable, whether or not it was obtained from the manager. If you sign on with a so-so manager, you could be working to pay commissions, which is not helping your career. Be sure that reasonable services are performed by the manager on your behalf in exchange for any compensation.

Who really uses managers? High profile stars and talent who are already successful find managers necessary. A good manager is like a financial planner. You only really need them when you have a large investment. When you are just beginning, most established managers are not interested in you. Be careful of managers who are interested in you if you have no screen credits. Promises come easy. There are NO guarantees in this business. Talk to your attorney before signing anything.

Over the years , I have been approached by many people who wanted to manage my career. None of these proposed "managers" was ever able to indicate to me that they could help me achieve my goals, despite their excitement, big ideas, and promises. In other words, it was apparent to me that I would still do all the work and have the opportunity to pay them a commission for being "my manager." Fortunately, although I was often tempted, I never hired a manager. I found that I was always my best adviser. Most of the successful talent that I know have all worked without the assistance of a manger. My recommendation is this: if you are reading this book you definitely do not need a manager. Get an agent. Become a big fish in a small pond. When the sharks start swarming, get some advice, and then decide whether to jump in the ocean.

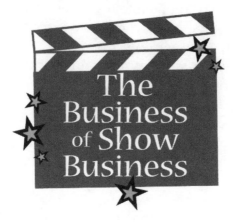

Chapter 9

Casting Directors

"Anything worth doing takes a risk....go out on that limb, that's where the fruit is!"

What is a Casting Director?

Casting directors are clients of the agents and of the production companies. The process of booking a job goes something like this:

Apple Computers wants a commercial. They contact their advertising agency who comes up with a concept and contracts with a production company to shoot the commercial. The ad agency or production company contacts a casting director to audition the correct types of talent. The casting director contacts talent agencies as well as sometimes contacting known actors directly. Sometimes the casting director asks agents to submit photos, sometimes the casting director asks for specific names. Although agents make recommendations and sometimes go to bat for talent, it is the casting directors who hold the power of whom they will put on tape and which talent will meet the agency executives who make the final decisions. I have known casting directors who erased an actors performance from the tape just because the casting director did not like the personality of the actor. This may seem unethical, but the casting director holds the cards. Be professional and be nice. Casting directors get to know talent from workshops, previous auditions, and completed jobs. Talent can improve their odds by "dropping by" a casting office to update photos. Sometimes a casting may be held for which you may be submitted. Be eager without being demanding and obnoxious.

If you have a talent agent, all casting directors need to know who that is. The name of your agent must be on your head shot, resume, and statistic sheet so the agent can be called. However, don't let the lack of an agent stop you from contacting casting directors. Most casting directors will keep a file of non-represented talent, especially if that talent is interested in working as an extra. Send 5 to 7 head shots with resumes, a statistic sheet with a current snapshot, a SASE for any application form that is necessary, and a short cover letter explaining that you are available for work and interested in registering with their casting service. Recently, many casting agencies are operating on-line database to eliminate keeping head shots on file. This requires you to visit the office in person, sit down at a computer and fill out the appropriate forms, have a digital photo shot of you, and sometimes pay a registration fee of no more than $20. (I indicate the maximum charge that I am aware of for legitimate casting services to distinguish them from the scams who regularly charge monthly, or fees of hundreds of dollars. Union members never are required to pay a casting fee…another benefit of being a union member) Please note: casting directors are required to have a normal business license if they are independent. They are not franchised by the unions, therefore the unions do not have any jurisdiction over their legitimacy. The Casting Society of America is a professional organization of casting directors that was formed to raise the visibility of the profession and provide a forum for its members. Membership is not automatic; members must apply and meet certain criteria. Commercial casting directors have a separate organization. CSA activities include working with minority and disadvantaged actors; workshops, and providing a communications link with the Association of Talent Agents. It is normal for casting companies to ask for a small up front filing fee of $10 to $20 per person for non-union, non-represented talent. This fee is waived for all union talent and agency representation, and in some instances for children.

Cautionary note: Sometimes you will read in the papers or trades that a showcase is being held where many casting directors will be in attendance. BEWARE! Many of these so called "talent showcases" charge high fees for a performance which may be useless to you in reaching the appropriate casting people. Keep in mind that anyone can call himself a casting director. It's your responsibility to make sure the casting person is legitimately employed in the entertainment field. Because casting directors are not governed by our performing union contracts, scams do exist. Unfortunately, many casting people make a great deal of their income by offering photography sessions, acting classes, and talent showcases. Some services may be excellent, many are worthless. Actors often feel compelled to hire the casting person for their head shots or to coach them in the hopes of being offered auditions. Don't fall into that trap. Only use the additional services of a casting person if you are convinced that what is being offered is valuable to your career. Often I have witnessed new actors take classes from a casting person only to be scorned by the casting office and never called in to audition. I also have seen horrible photos shot by a casting director/ photographer which were rejected by the agent, and once again, the actor is "blackballed" and not summoned to audition at that casting office. Most legitimate casting professionals are just that...professional, but it is always wise to check with your fellow actors, your agent, and the unions before engaging in activities that are going to cost you money and perhaps your career. Do your homework to discover if the services offered are worth your time, effort, and hard earned dollars.

Frequently asked questions of casting directors

1. What qualities are necessary to impress the casting director?

   The most important quality is to be right for the role. Auditioning is subjective and casting people often trust their gut instinct. It is important to have a professional attitude, good training, and to come looking like the role. You don't have to impress anyone. Rely on self-confidence and talent. If you don't get cast today, you may be cast another day.

2. If I gave a bad audition, can I try again?

   Sometimes a casting director will allow you to do a different reading if they are not running behind schedule. It is best to ask them if you may read again and not demand that you read again. Casting directors want you to book the role so that they don't have to audition hundreds of actors. Most of all, do the best job you can the first time around. If you have done your warm-up exercises and really rehearsed your role, you should be prepared. Always arrive at least 15 minutes in advance of your audition so that you will have enough time to read over the script. Doing a cold reading "stone cold" is not a good choice. It's better to let another actor go ahead of you to allow yourself a couple of minutes to prepare.

3. Once a role is cast, are auditions still held?

Not usually. Once a role has been cast, offices move on to the next role. There is not enough time to keep running auditions when a good actor has already been chosen.

4. Do casting directors accept submissions from talent who do not have an agent?

Yes, although most casting directors prefer to work with agents they like and trust. It is always good to submit your head shots and resumes at the beginning of your career and then keep the casting personnel updated as you grow and change. Don't send videotapes, however, unless requested to do so.

5. Does the casting director have the final decision in the casting process?

Sometimes yes but usually no. Most often, the casting director will present a list of first choices to the director or advertising director who will make the final decision. Never take anything you hear in the casting office as an offer of employment unless you have been told point blank: "You have the job."

6. Will casting directors from other cities call me in if I submit my photos to them?

Because our industry is so fast paced and decisions are made sometimes only a few hours before shooting, it is best to live in the city in which you want to work. Many San Francisco actors try to commute to Los Angeles for work. Agents and casting people will audition you, but it can become very costly for the actor. Production companies do not pick up your travel tabs if you are from out of town. If you are traveling to a city where you plan on visiting for an extended stay, by all means let the casting people know of your availability.

7. Is it better to stand or sit during a reading?

An audition is your time and you need to do whatever the role and your comfort level decide. If you have a choice, I suggest standing as people generally exude more energy and personality when standing than when sitting. However, if you are being videotaped, it is best to inquire if you can move around. Don't rearrange the furniture and don't touch the casting person.

8. What is the most important tool an actor has besides talent?

An actors head shot is the most important tool as very often an audition is arranged by head shots first. A head shot must look like you. A misleading photo costs more than one lost audition. Don't waste time by sending bad or outdated photographs. For example, a pile of head shots are delivered to the casting office. The casting directors make two piles: 'yes' to come for the audition and 'no', not this time. We never know why we are rejected or accepted. Sometimes it has to do with matching up families. A head shot must "speak" to the auditioner. There must be something that sets you apart, that creates an inner life. Casting people look at several hundred photos a day...would yours interest them?

9. Is it a good idea to say "I really need this job?"

Desperation is not attractive. Having self-confidence and talent says you are a winner. Obviously you want the job or you would not be on the audition. If you NEED the audition, you should not be on the audition. Respect yourself, be professional and prepared. If you really love and use the product for which you are auditioning, it is legitimate to say so, but don't go overboard.

In summary, the casting directors are your allies. If you are talented and professional, you make them and your agent look good. They will then call you in repeatedly. Many casting directors also book background talent. They are looking for versatile, easy-going talent who want to be extras. If you have a large wardrobe, transportation, and are flexible, dependable, on time and easy to work with, the same casting company will probably call you directly often. As with anything, the best way to make yourself invaluable is to be punctual, professional and be prepared. The triple "P"'s, as I call it.

For a list of approved casting agencies in your area, contact your local SAG or AFTRA office. Your franchised talent agency should also be able to provide you with a recommended list. You may be asked to send a SASE or to pay a small fee for this listing.

For all casting agencies, mail a current photo and resume with a cover letter saying whether you are S.A.G., or A.F.T.R.A., and whether you are interested in working as an extra on a project. Make sure you include your phone number. You would be amazed at the number of submissions both agents and casting directors receive with no contact information. Send a SASE envelope for any application or information they wish to send you. Do not telephone these casting directors unless they contact you. Many of the casting agencies have special phone lines with recorded messages explaining how to submit information, stating what projects are currently being cast, or giving the hours or operation. Feel free to use these recorded message phone lines to keep current with what is going on in the city in which you want to work.

Casting Sheet Example

A sheet similar to this will be given to you to be filled out for each audition and returned to the sign-in desk with a photo and resume. You usually need to fill out two similar forms BEFORE auditioning, so allow enough time for yourself. A Polaroid or digital photo is usually taken at the audition and stapled to the right of your name and statistics.

Note: Be sure your sizes are correct, that you do NOT write your Social Security number, even if asked, and that you are available on shoot dates.

Starmaker Casting Company

NAME_____

ADDRESS_____

HOME PHONE_____SERVICE_____

WORK PHONE_____OTHER PHONE_____

AGENT_____AGENT'S PHONE_____

UNIONS____SAG_____AFTRA_____AEA_____

SOCIAL SECURITY NUMBER_____

(AUTHOR'S NOTE: NEVER GIVE THIS OUT UNLESS BOOKED ON THE JOB)

HEIGHT_____WEIGHT_____HAIR_____EYES_____

ETHNICITY_____

AGE OF MINOR_____BIRTHDATE (IF UNDER 18)_____

DOES MINOR HAVE A VALID WORK PERMIT?_____

WOMEN SIZES:

SKIRT_____HAT_____BLOUSE____SHOE____DRESS_____

PANTS_____GLOVE_____RING_____INSEAM_____

SLEEVE_____BUST_____WAIST_____HIPS_____

MEN SIZES:

COAT____SHIRT/NECK____SLEEVE_____HAT____

WAIST____INSEAM____SHOE____GLOVE____RING____

TODAY'S DATE_____

ARE YOU AVAILABLE TO DO EXTRA WORK?_____

(NOTE: I feel it is a good idea to have these sizes and information written and updated monthly in your weekly planner and carried with you to all auditions. It is also a good idea to be available for extra work if you are willing to do so...you never know if you will get "bumped" up or upgraded to a principal performer.)

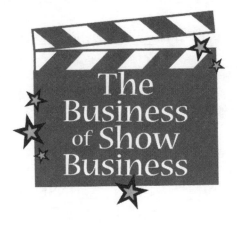

Chapter 10

Who's Who at Auditions

"Whether you think you can or think you can't...you're right."

Henry Ford

There are numerous people involved in the creation of an audition. The most important criteria for an actor is to always give an incredible performance no matter who is or is not in the room.

Casting Director

You may never meet anyone other than the casting director at an audition these days because of the use of video playback machines. The casting director is your friend. He or she likes you. You would not be at this audition if the casting person did not think you were right for the part. The casting director is usually hired by the advertising agency or production agency to find the talent.

The Advertising Agency

The advertising agency producer is in charge of the commercial. He/she probably has a casting director or director that saw your photograph in the first place and asked for you to be sent in. Maybe your agent sent in a package that contained your headshot. The producer or director of the project is sometimes present at auditions and call-backs. You may have the opportunity to meet the copywriter, art director, and some assistants.

The Client

The client is the company who produces or makes the product, for example, Apple Computers, Coca Cola, Clairol, or Ford Motor Company. The client hires the advertising agency to produce the commercial. Sometimes the account executive from the company is at the audition and might have some decision in who gets the part.

To whom should you read?

All these people are important in the final selection for the commercial. Which person has more say differs with each production. In reality, it doesn't matter who is the most important. What is important is your reading. If in doubt, ask to whom you should give your audition. For general rules of thumb, if you are being video-taped make eye contact with the camera. If it is a personal interview, be pleasant and relaxed with everyone. Smile and read to the friendliest person or whomever makes you feel most welcomed. Believe in yourself and your abilities. Want the job enough to know that you are good enough to have it, and you may just get it.

The interview

A resume is just words on paper but an interview gives you the opportunity to divulge your real personality, show the real you. Concern yourself only with giving your most excellent performance. You may not be chosen for this job because you are too pretty, too ugly, too blond, too brunette, too tall, too skinny, too young, too old; but if you leave a good impression, the casting director, the advertising agency, the client, or the producer may call you in for something else at another time. We can't be right for every job. In the end, winners win because they believe in themselves and never give up. Do your best. Hang in there and keep on trying!

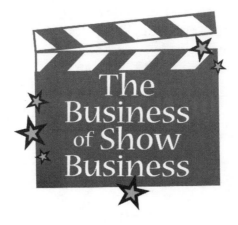

Chapter 11

The Audition or Interview...
Important Tips

"Without challenge, there is no achievement."

1. Know where you are going, the exact address, phone number (in case you get lost), what commercial or part you are reading for and who you are to see. Get the time to be there and allow 15 extra minutes and ask how you are to dress of if you are to bring extra wardrobe. It's a good idea to buy a good map of the area so you won't get lost. Don't wear perfumes, after shaves, or any scents.

2. Before you go in the door, get yourself together. Take a deep cleansing breath and relax. Check

your clothing, hair, and face. Make sure you have a couple copies of your photo and resume with you. Exercise your vocal chords a bit so you won't be squeaky. Do you feel good? Great, open the door, go in and smile! First impressions are the most important and remember you never get a second chance at a first impression!

3. Look for the sign-in sheet. Always sign in. It requires your name, the agent who sent you on the audition, and your actual call time as well as time you arrived. Although you are asked for your social security number, don't give it until you are booked on the job. In these technological days, don't give out your social security casually. If you don't have a social security number, get one. You can not work without one.

4. Ask if there is copy to read. Copy is a script. If not, there may be a storyboard which are pictures/drawings you can study that will give you some idea of what the client is trying to do with this commercial.

5. Find a quiet corner and read the copy over several times. Don't use this time to talk to old friends. You are here to try to get the job. Work at it. Do your script analysis. All commercials are conversational. Personalize the script. Remember the four important questions: Who am I? Who am I talking to? Why am I here? Where am I going? Go ahead and mark your script. Fold your script as small as possible and practice. Rehearse, rehearse, rehearse.

6. Your name is called. Take a deep breath. Relax, let out all the tension and stress. Smile and walk into the room. If a hand is offered for you to

shake, be personal and shake the hand. If not, go directly to your mark and prepare to do your reading.

7. The mark is the X or T or tape on the floor or wherever the casting director asks you to stand. Take directions from him or her. Feel free to ask how tight the camera will be on you...close up, medium shot, or full length.

8. Make eye contact with your friend, the camera. Start in your mind your conversation with your friend, the camera.

9. When told to slate, say your name only in an enthusiastic but real way. If asked a question, answer truthfully. Slate with glasses and hats off, if you wear them.

10. Take a second after slating, then go directly into the commercial. You have the first and last lines completely memorized and by now you should be able to do a cold reading with the rest. Be personal, professional, friendly and REAL. Don't sell, just talk to your friend and be conversational. Know that the casting person wants you to get the job. Make eye contact and interact with the camera. Do not physically touch anyone. Hold your script, even though you may have it memorized. It is best that the casting person knows this is a work in progress, not the finished product. Keep props to a minimum.

11. End your commercial with a smile, nod, shrug...what is called a button. Make it clean and simple. If asked to read again, be creative, listen to directions, and go with it. Be positive. You can do it!

12. Don't make any negative comments or chide yourself. Keep your personality going until the tape machine has stopped and you have said "thank you" and left the room.

13. Sign out the correct time you finished. Gather your belongings and leave still smiling. Don't make any comments on how you think you did until you're far away from the building. The fact is, you really don't know how well you did so don't judge yourself. Be happy.

14. Keep smiling and enjoy the rest of your day. Do something fun and forget about the audition. It was just another experience in life. Relax.

15. If you get a call-back, which means you go to perform again, this time usually for the clients as well as the video, be happy. Relax, they like you.

16. Find out all the information again as listed in number one. Go dressed EXACTLY as you were in the original audition unless told otherwise by your agent. You'll probably be asked to do the same script as before, so if you remember it, learn it well. Be prepared to talk to real people this time so have great answers to "Tell me about yourself." Give variances in your script if asked.

17. Remember that acting is reacting. Never become a character. Vanessa Redgrave said: "I do not identify with the character. I identify the character." Go for it!

18. After the audition and callbacks, forget about it. Do something nice for yourself, go get ice cream, take a walk, enjoy a movie. Don't call anyone to ask if you got the role, it you did, you'll be contacted.

19. Use the time between auditions to practice your craft. Take classes, get a camcorder and video tape yourself, read books on the craft of acting. Keep your life going, keep interesting and have fun!

Keep Smiling! Good Luck...You can do it!

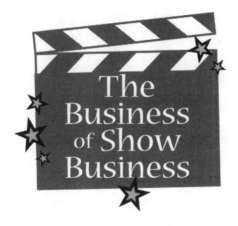

Chapter 12

Scripts and Scenes

"Imagination is more important than facts."
Albert Einstein

Structure of a Scene

1. Exposition-introduces the character, setting, time, situation, etc.
2. Rising Action-a series of incidents and events leading to the conflict.
3. Conflict-the struggle between opposing forces. The tensions between man versus nature, society, etc.
4. Climax-the highest point of tension in the scene.
5. Falling Action-a series of incidents and events leading to the resolution.

6. Denouement-the final resolution

Analyze a Commercial Script

Commercials are very well-planned pieces of material whose sole function is to sell a product or service. Most commercials have the same format: PROBLEM, SOLUTION, RESOLUTION. They usually begin with a "Grabber" or attention seeker and have a closing slogan. The actor's job is to discover the best way to sell the commercial without seeming like selling. Because the purpose is to sell, a commercial contains all the points of a good sales pitch:

1. The Gimmick: "I've got major news!" (attention grab)

2. The Problem: "We've seen a lot of new soft drinks, the same old flavors with different labels."

3. The Solution: "Finally a soft drink to get excited about...Caprio Guarana!" (Solution is usually the name of the product)

4. The Rational: "Caprio has a totally new and refreshing taste." (Rationale explains why the product is better than everything else)

5. The Resolution: "It's natural, caffeine-free, and (she takes a drink) " (Resolution tells how the product will improve your life, make you feel better, usually has the actor buying or using the product being very happy)

6. The Closing Slogan: "It's delicious...um, Caprio, available at your local store." (Closing is asking for you to purchase it. May give names of store that will carry this product.)

Look for key words and phrases. Try to approach each section with a different mood. Be innovative, be original, go out on a limb, take a risk with your delivery and your performance. Remember to sell yourself and the product will sell itself.

Commercial Script Steps

1. Read through the script several times.
2. Put it in your own words making sense out of it. Understand it, make it your own personal experience.
3. Know who you are, to whom you are speaking, where are you going, and why are you here?
4. All commercials are conversational. Be real. Have beat changes and mood transitions as in real conversation. Bring it to humanity. Confessions, secrets, personal pointers all work well.
5. Fold your copy to the smallest possible size.
6. Mark your beats with a pencil and highlight your lines with a yellow or pink marker. Be creative and imaginative with your choices.
7. If you don't understand a word or can't pronounce a word, ASK...don't mispronounce the word, especially the product on the audition.
8. Visualize what you are saying. Physicalize (use physical actions) For example, words like ouch, stinky, scrumptious, etc.) Don't indicate or suggest. Surprise!
9. ALWAYS MEMORIZE THE FIRST AND LAST LINES.
10. Make eye contact with your friend, the camera.
11. Get their attention with your opening, keep building to the climax and after the denouement (final

resolution), button with something that comes naturally such as a laugh, smile, shrug, wink, etc.

12. All commercials end happily ever after.....

13. If you have no dialog in a commercial, remember to stay in the scene. Stay alive. Acting is good re acting. Physicalize more, but don't indicate.

Simple Script Breakdown

1. Read the script over several times and look at story board if one is available.

2. Memorize the first and last lines (a MUST) and more if you are able.

3. Believe what you are saying. Make it real.

4. Be natural.

5. Sell Yourself, not the product. Be yourself, be positive.

Easy Cold Reading Technique

1. Fold your copy.

2. Left thumb on left side of page.

3. Look down.

4. Mumble through the line, get a group thought.

5. Look up and make eye contact.

6. Complete the line and deliver to camera. Do not look down to next line until you have finished the first line. No slurring. Speak to the camera.

Chapter 13

Monologues

"Be glad of life because it gives you the chance to love and to work and to play and to look up at the stars."

Henry Van Dyke

A monologue is a scene in which only one person is speaking. Compelling monologues are useful audition tools, used more often for stage or agency auditions than for film and TV. When you choose a monologue, it is best to find material that has a character for which you could be cast and will showcase your skills to your best advantage. No point in trying to play a 50 year old man if you are 13 and a girl. You won't be cast in the role no matter how great you are, so choose something age and gender appropriate. Unless you are superb at accents or dialects, stay away from them. Don't choose a monologue from a famous play or movie as it is a no win situation. Two of the most common monologues are from "Streetcar named Desire" and "Cat on a Hot Tin Roof". Not only are agents and directors sick of seeing them, but if you perform like the stars you are considered a copy cat, if you do it differently, you'll be told you've chosen the wrong interpretation. Find something, new, fresh, different. I'm often asked about the monologue books available for actors. Mostly the monologues from these books are over used, however, the play that the monologue came from may be fresh and have a perfectly suitable additional monologue for you. My advice is to read the original play in total and see what you can find. If you can identify with a character, you could have a strong monologue. You don't ever want to choose a piece that makes you feel uncomfortable. Sometimes a story well told is fine. You don't need props, costuming, sound effects or music. Your voice and your body are your tools. You are auditioning to be seen and heard, not to hide under props. The piece needs to be self-explanatory with a minimum of words to set the scene.

It should be noted that rarely are monologues asked for in commercial or even film auditions. From my experience and that of my clients, it is usually agents who are interested in seeing a monologue performed before deciding on whether to represent a particular talent or not. Monologues are always used for stage production casting calls and sometimes for other castings, but only occasionally in the film/TV end of the business. Nevertheless, it is always a great idea to have a monologue ready and waiting for any opportunity to perform. Practice, practice, practice and be prepared.

Relax, be prepared, and be interesting. Try not to indicate or physicalize too much. Let the words flow naturally as if this was the first time you said them. Be present in the scene, remember who you are, where you are, who you are talking to and where this is leading. Maintain your acting integrity by using common sense.

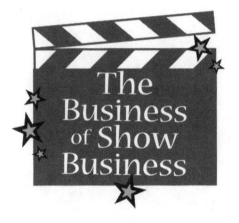

Chapter 14

Terms Written on Scripts

*"Worse than not having sight is
not having vision."*

Helen Keller

AUDIO: the sound portion, i.e. what we hear, words said

VIDEO: the on-camera portion, i.e. what we see, the action

V.O.: Voice over; off-camera person's voice. Radio commercials are all voice overs. Announcers who are not seen on the TV commercial are voice overs.

O.C.: On-camera, i.e. this is what will be seen.

CUT: When a scene changes to another scene or ends

DISSOLVE: Abbreviated as DISS; is when a scene blends into another scene

CU: Close-up

TCU: Tight Close-up

ECU: Extreme Close-up

MCU: Medium Close-Up

LS: Long Shot

WA: Wide Angle

SFX: Special Effects

INT: Interior

EXT: Exterior

ALT: Alternate shot; other scene or words

LOGO: Produce slogan or name

SUPER: Superimpose

MOS: Silent or no sound

TWO SHOT: Two people in one shot

Chapter 15

Who's Who on a Set

"The meeting of two personalities is like the product of two substances. If there is any reaction, both are transformed."

Carl Jung

When you see the credits roll at the end of a movie, have you ever wondered "what's a Best Boy or an ADR mixer"? Here is a brief glossary to help you understand who all those people are you will be working with.

EXECUTIVE PRODUCER: is usually the person who financed or got the financing for the film. Executive producers aren't usually involved in daily production decisions.

PRODUCER: is the person in charge of everything for a production. The producer does all the administrative and hiring jobs, signs up the director and big stars and may be the one who gets the financing. The producer is the person that gets the film into production and oversees all the logistics during pre and post postproductions.

DIRECTOR: in charge of overseeing all the creative aspects of the film working closely with writers, actors, production team and director of photography. Directors usually have their own style or flair which is recognizable in a film.

LINE PRODUCER/PRODUCTION MANAGER: in charge of the daily managing of the production. Reports to the producer and director.

DIRECTOR OF PHOTOGRAPHY: this person designs the lighting, frames the shots and directs the camera moves all based on the director's vision.

CASTING DIRECTOR: person responsible for finding the actors for the director and producer to interview.

SECOND UNIT DIRECTOR: Shoots footage, usually of backgrounds, or shots that will be added to the film. Shoots in the same style as directed by the director.

CAMERA OPERATOR: this person takes directions from the DP and runs the camera.

DOLLY GRIP: operates the dolly which is a piece of equipment on four wheels that allows the camera to move on a track. The dolly grip pushes the camera for the camera operator.

FOCUS PULLER: when actors move closer to the camera or move further away, the focus puller refocuses the lens of the camera.

LOCATION MANAGER: this location scout finds the best places to shoot and arranges for permits.

PRODUCTION DESIGNER: supervises the visuals of the film, designing sets, choosing furnishings, accessories, colors, creating the overall theme.

SET DECORATOR: usually a trained interior designer who purchases or rents the furnishings based on the production designers advice.

LEAD PERSON: this is the assistant set director who is in charge of purchasing materials to decorate the set. Works with the set decorator and production designer.

STUNT COORDINATOR: choreographs each stunt, making sure safety is first.

SOUND DESIGNER: in charge of all audio on the film

SOUND MIXER: head of on-location sound recording team including boom operator and third man.

SOUND EFFECTS EDITOR: enhances and designs the sound in post-production.

BOOM OPERATOR: uses a long adjustable pole with a microphone at the end holding it close enough to get the right sound without being in the shot.

THIRD MAN: is a cable handler, handling everything related to sound.

SCRIPT SUPERVISOR: enables continuity by making sure that the same lines are used with the same physical gestures from various angles of the scene.

ADR: ADR means "additional dialogue recording." The ADR mixer works with actors to dub dialogue in post production (also called "looping"). The director may choose to be present during an ADR session. The ADR supervisor works directly with the director to find scenes that will need dubbing.

FOLEY ARTIST: makes sound effects in post production by using various materials and props to simulate certain sounds.

GAFFER: set ups the lights under the directors or director of photography's directions. Sometimes designs the lighting.

BEST BOY: this is the Gaffer's assistant who supervises the lighting crew, orders lighting equipment.

GRIP: works with different types of lighting equipment, setting up lamps and diffusion material.

ELECTRICIAN: in charge of finding the electricity or maintaining a generator.

STAND BY PAINTER: touches up objects within a scene to prevent unwanted reflections or colors during shooting.

EDITOR: works closely with the director to edit the footage.

PUBLICIST: publicity person, writing articles, arranging interviews.

Chapter 16

On Professionalism

"The evasion of failure is not the same thing as the quest for success."

The difference between an amateur and a professional is the way in which you conduct yourself. If you want to be a success, you must have your "act" together. Stop complaining that "your agent" is not doing enough for you and examine your own strengths and weaknesses. How much excess baggage are you carrying around?

Ask yourself these questions:

★ Am I afraid of success?

★ Am I afraid of failure?

☆Do I look at auditions as an opportunity or a nuisance?

☆ Do I feel powerful or manipulated?

☆ Do I feel all casting people are against me?

☆ Am I worth selling?

☆ Can I sell myself?

☆ What am I doing to improve my craft?

☆ Is my resume updated?

☆ Does my body language indicate confidence or fear?

☆ Am I using new photos, or ones that don't look like me now?

☆ Am I always prepared?

☆ Am I a winner?

Only you can determine your future. You can be successful and have anything you desire if you are willing to put in the time, effort, and expense to get it. Success is not handed out on a silver platter. I don't believe in luck, I believe in working the system. My Los Angeles agent once told me that what was needed to succeed in this industry was tenacity, perseverance, and talent....in that order. Therefore luck is determination combined with hard work and perseverance. To be a professional, be organized, well-groomed, versatile and flexible. Eliminate fear or use your fear to your advantage to open the doors of success. The amount of effort you put into your career is directly related to the amount of success you will achieve. Review your work and improve upon it. Progress daily and act immediately. Learn to handle frustrations and disappoint-ments as they will surely occur just as the sun rises. Always know it is NOT you the "personal" you that is being rejected. Create new challenges and goals. Learn something new everyday. Read books, go to plays, see musicals, participate in productions. Don't sit by the phone and wait. No one is going to knock on your door and offer to make you a star. You already are the star of your own performance, so get out there and show someone. Stop blaming and complaining…just take action to get reaction. You can do it. Sure it is scary, nerve wracking, and sets you up for constant rejection, but if you want guarantees and stability, don't choose acting as your career. You make the impossible possible. YOU!

<u>Grow, take charge, be responsible and your dreams will come true.</u>

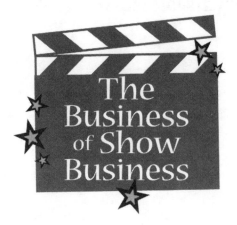

Chapter 17

Photography

"Happiness begins in your soul and shines through your eyes."

In show business, the adage goes, "you are only as good as your worst photograph." Head shots are our calling cards, one of the most important sales tools we possess. So it is understandable that actors must find the right photographer to shoot the best photo and capture the inner spirit of the actor...a photo that transmits personality, emotion, and depth. Getting a great shot is not the rarity if you know which photographers are creative professionals in our industry. Start planning your photo shoot well in advance of when you really need them. Know that from the day you shoot until you actually are holding head shots that can be distributed is probably a minimum of 6 to 8 weeks. If you are just starting out, getting a black and white head shot and a 3/4 body shot are the way to go. Plan your wardrobe so that no two finished shots will have the same clothing in them. Stay away from plaids, stripes, flowers, and bold exotic designs. You want to be simple, straight-forward and able to convey a variety of looks. Think "middle America" as a great look. For kids, "off the playground" fresh, perky, and youthful is the best choice. Find a photographer by asking your acting coach, agent, or acting colleagues. Keep in mind that SAG and AFTRA franchised agents, because of their contract with the unions, may NOT demand that you use a particular photographer. They may offer suggestions, tell you whose work gets talent the most jobs, give you a list of recommended photo-graphers, show you photos that convey the subject well, but it is ultimately up to you to find the appropriate photographer for you. Don't go to the yellow pages as acting/modeling photography is very different than straight studio or wedding portraits. A head shot is NOT a glamour shot, nor is it a sexy pose. It is a personality shot capturing the way you look every day…warm, friendly, and saleable…like a charming next door neighbor.

You hire the photographer so you have the right to ask lots of questions. Here are questions that need to be asked of the potential photographer:

☆ Does the photographer specialize in acting/ modeling photos?

☆ What local agents work with the photographer?

☆ How many rolls will be shot?

☆ Who will keep the negatives?

☆ What is included in the price (for example a contact sheet, make-up and hair styling, 8 x 10 copies)?

☆ How long will the session take?

☆ Will Polaroids or digitals be used to set up the shots?

☆ What kind of wardrobe should be brought on the shoot?

☆ What is the re-shoot policy if you are not happy with your photo session?

☆ May I see a portfolio of former photo sessions?

Make sure you have a lively telephone rapport. It is important that you have faith in his experience. If you wish more clarification of the work, ask to set up an appointment to see the photographer's portfolio. Some photographers are too busy to do this, so if it is a photographer recommended by someone you trust, ask your friend to show you their head shot done by that particular person and quiz that person about the experience. Agents also keep head shots shot by a variety of recommended photographers in their offices. Once you have hired the photographer, discuss wardrobe, make-up and hair. My suggestion is to always bring lots of clothing and let the photographer help you select the items. Make sure everything is pressed and clean. Many photographers charge an extra fee for make-up application anywhere from $75-$150. Make-up for men is usually less. It is good to remember that you want your head shots to look as much like you as possible. As of this writing, a simple black and white head shot or 3/4 body shot with one roll of 36 exposures and two to three wardrobe changes costs in the range of $125 to $275. Expect to pay extra for each additional role of film, and sometimes per outfit change. A composite shoot costs more, usually $225 on up depending on the amount of looks. Prices vary greatly on location. Los Angeles appears to have the least expensive photographic sessions that I have seen, probably because it also has more actors and photographers than any other city in America. Competition always drives the price lower.

A composite is often used for commercial print jobs. A composite includes a head shot plus four or more action shots in a variety of locations with diversified wardrobe. A zed card, which is used for fashion work, is usually in color which costs more. However most models like to use copies of their "tear sheets" on their zed cards, so not as many new fashion looks need to be shot. In all scenarios, discuss fees with the individual photographer up front as photographers set their own rates for their varied services. Payment is usually 50% at time of shooting, with the balance when photos are complete.

Cancellation policies also differ, but 24 hours is standard. Obviously if you are ill, it is not wise to do a shoot. All legitimate photographers guarantee their work so if an agent is not happy with the contact sheet a re-shoot at no charge is in order. (Re-shooting to get different wardrobe, hairstyle, make-up or looks is not included in a free re-shoot). Show up for your session well rested and prepared for the shoot. I suggest doing acting warm-ups to relax and focus your energy. Don't expect the photographer to do all the work, offer suggestions. Be spontaneous, have fun, relax and you'll get a great shot. The ideal is not a perfect photo but a photo that presents you in a positive light...that reaches out and grabs people.

What to Do after the Photo Shoot

Your photo shoot was successful, you are now looking at a positively wonderful contact sheet. What's the next step? If you have an agent, call the agent and ask if the agent is willing to look at the contact sheet and help you select your best photos. If you are working with a coach, he or she has the expertise to help you through this process.

Whatever you do, don't choose the photos yourself. Parents see their beloved offspring differently than a casting person will. Your agent or coach know what the current looks are and what's hot. They want you to be successful so trust their input. If your photographer does not print up the original, you will need to go to a photo lab. My recommendation is to use only professional photo labs that deal with head shots and professional photographers. If you are working with black and white photos, go to a black and white specialty lab. No offense against the quick labs on your neighborhood corner, but honestly, you will not get the best results at those places. Also, if a lab ruins your original negatives, you have no recourse but to pay for a re-shooting. I have had several clients try to save a few bucks by going to the cheapest place they could find, only to have negatives lost or destroyed. In the end, these clients ended up paying many more times what the original professional lab costs would have been. It may cost you a little more to go to a professional lab, but it is well worth the extra effort, time, hassle, and money to develop a high quality in focus photo.

After you have selected the best shots and have printed your 8 x 10's at a professional photo lab, you will need to formulate a layout. Again, you'll need some help. For duplication purposes, your 8 x 10's will be made into 8 1/2 x 11's with your name, union affiliation, and date of birth if you are under 18. At a duplication house you can get head shots in multiples of hundreds as well as business cards and postcards with your photo and statistical information imprinted. My favorite places are listed below but feel free to use your own duplication houses:

Exact photos and digital
1700 Bush Street #12
San Francisco, Ca.
415-567-0671

(takes photographs and negatives and enhances these images on a pre-press digital file which can then be sent to the companies listed below for press)

Duplication of head shots, composites, zed cards, postcards, etc.

(Prices vary, so contact each place for a price sheet)

Supershots
971 Goodrich Blvd.
Los Angeles 90022
(213) 724-4809

Anderson Graphics
P.O. Box 2427
Van Nuys 91401
(818) 786-5235

Quantity Photos
5432 Hollywood Blvd.
Hollywood
(213) 467-6178

ABC Pictures
1867 E. Florida
Springfield, Mo 65803-4583

Metro Disk
836 Harrison St.
San Francisco, 94107
415-836-9222

Once you have at least 100-300 head shots, you are ready to submit them to agents, casting directors and production companies. Make sure to keep your original 8 x 10 photos in a safe place in case you decide to want to create another head shot.

Chapter 18

Resumes

*"Thought is the blossom; language the bud;
action the fruit behind it."*
Ralph Waldo Emerson

After your head shot, the single most important calling card is your resume. Every resume must be current, accurate and honest. There is an established format used on both the East and West Coasts. This format has been approved by the Casting Society of America, the Association of Talent Agents and is the form generally used by actors nationwide. It is a standardized form familiar to producers, directors, and casting directors. Although each talent agency may vary slightly, it is best to write your initial resume following this one. Notice that there are no dates on an acting resume. Never lie on your resume about any work or training. In the beginning it is acceptable to put extra work on a resume but after principal work has been acquired, remove all extra material. This resume represents you. Print on good quality bond paper and staple to the back of head shots on 4 corners. You may also print your resume directly on the back of your head shot, but if you choose to do this it is advised to only print in small quantities. Hopefully you will need to update your resume regularly!

Standardized categories for size of roles are:

☆ Featured: any principal role, one liner on up.

☆ Co-Star: A substantial role, usually consisting of one or more meaty scenes and usually accompanied by "co-star" billing negotiated by your agent.

☆ Guest Star: used for TV only with credits negotiated by your agent.

☆ Recurring featured

☆ Recurring co-star

☆ Starring: lead role

☆ Host

Sample Resume

YOUR NAME (centered, big letters)

AGENT CONTACT:
(name of Agency; agent,
address phone) If no agent,
your service, pager, fax number

STATISTICS:
DOB (If under 18)
Hair: Ht. Size:
Eyes: Wt. Shoe:

UNIONS: (If you don't belong to a union, eliminate this category)

FILM:
Name of film   Role (guest, co-star, featured)   Director or Producer
(List all your films including student, industrials, etc. until you build credits)

TELEVISION:
Name of show   Role (guest, co-star, featured)   Director or Producer

THEATRE:
Title of Play   Role (List in order of best roles)   Name of Theatre

COMMERCIALS:
Updated list upon request or conflicts on request or if you have done hundreds write: "over 200 commercials, conflicts upon request"

TRAINING:
List all the acting, singing, dancing, voice, gymnastics, martial arts and musical instrument training, where and with whom.

SPECIAL SKILLS:
LANGUAGES: what you speak fluently
SPORTS: list all in which you are proficient. If it is not on here, you don't do it. Casting people are not mind readers.
SPECIAL ABILITIES: list everything else, i.e., computer training, ear wiggling, etc.

OTHER MEDIA: commercial model/actor/voice talent/hand model, etc. (This is where you list the other acting abilities that are not listed on resume.)

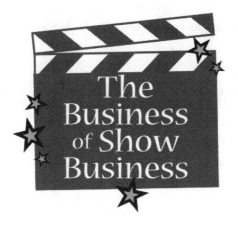

Chapter 19

Preparing for Your Success

"You will see it when you believe it."

You are the most important ingredient in your own success. Poet Miriam Viola Larsen wrote: "The world always steps aside for people who know where they are going." When you are passionate and dedicated, it shows. Enthusiasm is contagious.

Tom Clancy said: "Nothing is so real as a dream."

Luck is ability creating opportunity.

Our talents are gifts from God. It is our obligation and responsibility to share these talents with the world. This is not ego. This is doing what we were put on this earth to do. Share and service others. Entertain, amuse, and beguile.

Research shows that people do not become high performers by imitating others but by being themselves. High performance occurs when a person goes beyond their own expectations in ways that are unique to them, consistently and repeatedly. In other words, state your plan, then exceed it in every way. Proclaim your vision and your mission.

The Winning Attitude

You are what you think you are.

If you are happy, have a positive outlook and smile frequently, you'll find that others want and like to be around you. Others will smile because you have brought out a smile in them. Most people like "up" people. No one really wants to be around a loser. So act like a winner without being a preening peacock. In other words, leave the chip on your shoulder at home. Gaining a positive image of yourself is a simple process. With a little practice you can increase your self-esteem and develop a winning attitude.

Exercises for Success

Here are some suggestions and exercises to help you toward your goal of a positive self-image:

1. VISUALIZATION AND IMAGINATION

Practice using your imagination. Recall your favorite experiences in vivid detail. Concentrate on only the positive qualities. The human mind is a remarkable bio-computer capable of marvelous action. For example, the subconscious level of your mind cannot distinguish between real and imagined behavior. If you vividly imagine an action in your subconscious mind, your conscious level treats that action as if it really happened and it triggers your behavior towards achievement of that action. Sports figures use this type of imagination to visualize winning. We can alter this for success in any facet of our daily life.

2. LEARN TO LISTEN

When we are listening we always learn more about ourselves and those around us. We have 2 ears and 1 mouth so we should listen twice as much as we talk. Good actors are actors who listen well.

3. WRITE A GOAL RESUME

Write a short resume of your personal qualities. Include everything you like about yourself. (Your "How great I am" journal could help here) Then write a resume of your professional qualities. Concentrate on the present. Write a second resume concentrating on the future potential of your personal and professional qualities. Meld the two together to find your passionate goals and purpose. Read your new resume every week and visualize yourself exercising these positive traits. Keep upgrading and revising as needed.

4. ELIMINATE CLUTTER

Get rid of the confusion in your life. Clean out your closets of negative thoughts, actions, and acquaintances. Decide to allow only constructive alliances in your life. Open yourself to clear, positive thoughts and feelings. Rid yourself of the FEAR of success. Enjoy organized chaos!

5. BE A TERRIFIC PERSON

Concentrate your thoughts on what an original and unique person you are. You are special, you are different, you are the best at what you do. See yourself in this terrific and magnified light. Don't criticize or knock your abilities. Make the best better.

6. I AM A WINNER

Align yourself, your thinking and your actions with other winners. Friends mirror ourselves. Choose to be around forward thinking, upbeat people who are on the winning track. Know you are a winner. Apply the winning attitude to everything you do in life. Choose to be a winner and you will be one.

7. POSITIVE ATTITUDE

Always project a positive attitude towards your family, friends, and fellow actors. Positive actions, thoughts, attitudes create success and happiness. Be happy for the success of others. If they can do it, so can you. Your turn may be next. Enthusiasm is contagious.

8. DOWN AND OUT...SOMETIMES

There will be times when you are feeling down, depressed, overwhelmed, unloved, and ugly. All people experience this. Go with it, feel it, know it is part of your humanness. Give yourself a time limit, an hour, a day, a week to just feel these sad, negative emotions. Winners fail too, but winners don't stay down. A winner is not a whiner. Winners pop back up and get into the race. A winner remains optimistic even in the worst of times. It is a matter of learning to handle frustration and disappointment. When you are in the gutter the only place to go is up. Have a high opinion of your self-worth. If you blew the audition, learn from it, then forget it and go on. Don't dwell on "what could have been."

9. RESPONSIBILITY

Assume total responsibility for your actions. You are what you are what you are! When you make a mistake, admit it, apologize, fix it, and get on with it. Don't apologize for your successes. You deserve them, you've earned them.

10. HUGS AND KISSES

Share your love and appreciation with those who have helped you along the way. Show your spouse, children, and friends that you care for and about them. Say "I love you" often. Give lots of hugs and kisses. Most of all, love yourself and say "I love the me inside of me."

11. THE GOLDEN RULE

As often as it has been said, it is not practiced enough. Always do unto others as you want done unto you. Treat others fairly and with respect. It comes bounding back to you.

12. BE ALIVE

Celebrate your life, your health, your aliveness. There is no time to feel sorry for yourself. There is always some-one somewhere who is suffering more than you. Be happy that you are here in this body in this life in this time.

13. COMMUNICATE

The quality of your life is directly related to the quality of your communications. Develop rapport with others. Learn to handle frustrations and see others points of view. Validate others opinions. There are no rights or wrongs, just feelings and opinions and these are real. Communicate, validate, commiserate…don't dictate.

14. BELIEVE

Believe you can do anything, because you can. As we think, so shall we experience. What you think about, and talk about comes about. You can have it all, if your belief is strong enough, your vision is clear and you are willing to work to accomplish it. You deserve the best, treat yourself to self-esteem.

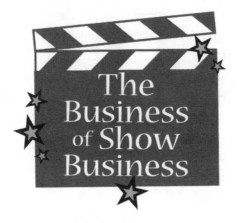

Chapter 20

What is Self Esteem?

"If you think you are beaten, you are.
If you think you dare not, you don't.
If you'd like to win, but think you can't,
it's almost a cinch, you won't.
Life's battles don't always go
to the stronger or faster man.
Sooner or later, the man who wins,
is the man who thinks he can."

Author unknown

Self-esteem is your feeling about yourself. It is the image you have of yourself—that picture of yourself that you carry around in your mind. A realistic self-image is important because you tend to behave as you believe yourself to be.

Self-image is formed through the messages received throughout a lifetime from parents, teachers, peers, and experiences. With high self-esteem, you can set positive goals for yourself. With high self-esteem, you will be able to take risks to achieve growth. With high self-esteem, you will be able to form loving relationships.

What can you do to build self-esteem? Start with yourself! Embrace challenges! The person who relishes challenges will be successful. Challenges don't represent a threat but an opportunity for problem solving. Look at the big picture to realize that your success or failure will be directly related to how well you meet and solve critical challenges.

Practice expressing your values, feelings, and opinions openly. Demonstrate by listening to others (especially children) that their values, feelings, opinions are of interest to you. Become aware of the abilities, talents and strengths that you possess. Point out to others their abilities, talents, and strengths. Give lots of compliments. Validate others.

Give yourself recognition for small positive changes in your life. Endorse others for small positive changes as well. Create an environment in which "building people up" is the norm, rather than "putting people down". Stop using "put down" statements completely, and eliminate the "blaming and complaining".

Smile! Have fun! Be wild and crazy!

Cynthia's Recipe for Success

©1998-2002

For a healthy body mind, and spirit....

Blend together generous amounts of

☆ spontaneity

☆ forgiveness

☆ giggles

☆ serendipity

☆ appreciation

☆ joy

☆ challenges

☆ integrity

☆ humor

☆ acceptance

Add walks on the beach, good books, piggy back rides with the kids, sunsets, the wild kingdom, mangoes and lemonade. Stir in smiling attacks, daydreaming, back rubs, angel dust, starlight, and sheer delight.

Bake for a lifetime while slowly topping with

☆ a quest for knowledge

☆ unconditional love

☆ freedom

☆ inspiration

☆ choices

☆ faith

☆ gratitude

☆ generosity

☆ prayer

It is normal for this recipe to encounter pain, sorrow, disappointment, discouragement, and dismay. It is not a failure. Every batch is special creating change, growth, and learning.

Serves one or a multitude with confidence, happiness and fulfillment of life's purpose.

Be prepared to share and cook up more!

Chapter 21

The Gift of Rejection

"Nee heb je, ja kan je krijgen." (You already have a no, you can always try for a yes)

"You're too tall, you're too short, you're too pretty, you're too ugly, you're too young, you're too old, your hair is too blonde, your hair isn't blonde enough, your eyes are too blue, your eyes need to be brown, you have too much experience, you're not experienced" How many times over that past twenty-six years of my acting career have I heard these words? There are not enough numbers in the universe!

Rejection is one of the most unpleasant words in the dictionary—refusals, repudiations, turn downs, rebuffs, renunciation, disapproval, snubbing—basically people are shouting "I don't want you! You're not good enough!"

And what have I done with all that rejection? I have made it part of my success strategies.

You are probably thinking I'm crazy to consider rejection a gift, but I can tell you from first hand experience that it is. From birth to death, we are going to be rejected thousands of times for one thing or another. It's a good idea to get used to it early on and learn to make rejection our friend.

When I was growing up, my parents instilled great confidence in me that I could do and be whatever I put my mind to. What I didn't realize was that other people were also putting their minds to similar things. This led to a lot of disappointment when I was runner-up instead of queen, or took second place in the talent contest or third place for my jar of jam at the fair. But none of this compared with the rejection that actors must learn to accept.

As an actor, every new day means interviewing for one or more new jobs. Sometimes weeks or months go by with every door slammed in our face.

Over the years, I have perfected the art of auditioning. I learn the script and prepare as best as possible. I dress for the part, I pump myself up, and I walk in that door knowing that I am a gift! Then I do the best audition I can possibly do on that day. I leave the room, refuse to replay the interview in my head, and go buy myself an ice cream to celebrate my achievement. If I get the job, it's icing on the cake. I'll celebrate again.

What I have always taught my acting students is to realize that it isn't "Cynthia, the person" who is being rejected. It is "Cynthia, the actor." As the actor, I probably am too tall, too short, too pretty, too ugly, too young, too old, too blonde, not blonde enough, too blue-eyed, too brown-eyed, too experienced, or not experienced enough. None of us can be right for every situation, every relationship, every job.

Most people are crushed by their first rejection but we have to get back up when we fall, falter, or fail, and turn our setbacks into comebacks. I tell my acting students that an actor is really hot if he lands one job for every thirty-six auditions. Life is the same. You may have to date thirty-five duds, look at thirty-five prospective homes, apply for thirty-five jobs. As hard as it is, try to see each "no" as tremendously positive because you are now just much closer to a "yes."

We won't get out of this world without experiencing lots of rejection sooner or later. The secret is to embrace it and never give up. Rejection is a numbers game. For every "no" we get, we are closer to a "yes"—but only if we keep going, keep giving, and keep improving. Yes, when you are feeling down and out, it's hard to get up and get going, but believe me, you can do it. Go for it, and keep going for it.

This is my favorite poem. I have it posted in my office, in my home, and have included it in all the books I have written. The author is anonymous, but this legacy is the best defense against rejection and being the star you are. I suggest you copy it and post it all over your home and office as well. As an actor or model, you will need to read it often.

Don't Quit

When things go wrong, as they sometimes will,
When the road you're trudging seems all up hill,
When the funds are low, and the debts are high,
And you want to smile, but you have to cry,
When care is pressing you down a bit,
Rest if you must, but don't you quit.

Life is queer with its twists and turns,
As everyone of us sometimes learns,
And many a failure turns about,
When he might have won had he stuck it out.
Don't give up though the pace seems slow,
You may succeed with another blow.

Success is failure turned inside out,
The silver tint of the clouds of doubt,
And you never can tell how close you are.
It may be near when it seems so far.
So stick to the fight when you're hardest hit.
It's when things seem worse,
That you must not quit.

If you think you are beaten, you are.
If you think you dare not, you don't.
If you'd like to win, but think you can't
It's almost a cinch that you won't.

For Life's battles don't always go
To the stronger or faster man.
But, sooner or later, the man who wins
Is the one who thinks he can.

—Anonymous

Success rarely comes on the first, second, third or fourth try. Sometimes even the hundredth. Keep trying and don't give up. Even when you are rejected unnecessarily, consider each rejection as character building. You are a miracle of life, and you can do it. Give yourself a break, but never quit. You are a star! Embrace each "no" and exclaim, "Thank you, I am now that much closer to a yes!"

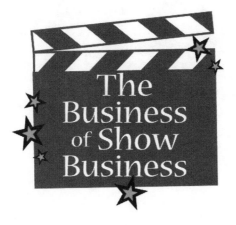

Chapter 22

Creativity, Language and Movement Exercises

"I am the captain of my soul.
I am the master of my fate"
William Henley

Fun and wild exercises to help you be the star you already are!

1. BELLY BREATHING, also known as *watermelon belly* or *baby breath*.

Learn to breathe properly by lying on the floor. Do not cross any part of your body as this stops the flow of energy. Make sure you are very comfortable. Put your right hand on the lower part of your stomach, right below your belly button. Inhale deeply through your nose, push the air to below your hand. This pushes your diaphragm in the air and feels like you have swallowed a watermelon. Hold for 20 seconds. Exhale slowly through your mouth. Do exercise three times in a row.

Babies until the age of about 2 1/2 breath normally from their diaphragms. That's what gives them the extended big bellies. This is the proper way to breathe. As we grow older, we tend to breathe very shallowly from our chests. In this way we cannot hold enough air to complete sentences and have stamina. Practice breathing. When you are good at this one, you can do it in your car or any time stressful situations arise. This exercise grounds and centers while relaxing our body, mind, and spirit.

2. THE MOAN

This is one of my favorite breathing exercises to help rid me of frustration and create harmony. Do the above belly breathing but on the exhale, let your breathe extend whatever sound comes out. Let the sound come from deep inside. Moan it out. Wow this feels good. Make sure to do it three times.

3. LION ROAR

Get on your haunches, curl your paws, and feel the power of the king of the jungle. Let it all out with a deep loud roar! BE THE LION!

4. COBRA SNAKE

Lie on the floor face down. Push up with your hands, like doing a push up. When you have reached full height, think of yourself as a slithering, slimy snake and hiss on the way down. Get in touch with ourselves at this lowest level. Now imagine the speed in the snake, and the softness of its skin and think of the snake as beautiful and necessary.

5. ENERGY SHAPE AND COLOR

Lie on your back, arms and legs outstretched. Do not cross any part of your body. Think of a color and a shape. Don't ponder, choose the first color and shape that comes to your mind. Now visualize this color and shape coming from the earth and working positive energy through every portion of your body...muscles, blood, nerves, etc. As you visualize, say out loud..."The purple star (substitute your own shape and color) is now revitalizing my feet, it is now at my ankles, it is rubbing my shins, it is now circling my knee...." and continue like this until the energy reaches the top of your head. It then goes out into the universe leaving you with this wonderful new energy.

6. MY GREATEST MOMENT

Do the above exercise, Color my World, then follow with three deep cleansing breaths. Shut your eyes and remember the most wonderful moment of your life. It can be anything from the time you were born despite your age now. Perhaps it was the first home run, a graduation, a good grade, the approval of someone you loved, or the birth of a child. It doesn't matter the significance to anyone else, only you. You must feel that moment...look around you and see all the people, how they are reacting to you, what the smells are, what time of day, what the area looked like. Memorize every detail. Delight in the wonderful feelings that you deserve. Now take this wonderful moment and record these same feelings into a time in the present day in which you want the same successful outcome. Visualize the same responses in this new situation. You are the star of the hour. Enjoy the sensations and decide this is the reaction you want from your actions. Make it happen.

7. STRETCH UP HIGH

Stand tall. Reach as high as you dare. Stand on your toes and reach for the stars. Now bend over and limply touch the ground. Stretch up, up, and up again, making a circle in the air. Sweep your arms around, jump up high off the ground. Which feels better? Do you want to reach and soar, or fall to the ground? Choice is always yours to make in life.

8. YAWN

The quickest way to get oxygen to your brain is to embrace a great big yawn. Stretch out your arms, open your mouth, and yawn. By faking it the first time, you'll begin a yawn. Suck in the air, let the eyes water, and yawn big.

9. FLY LIKE A BIRD

Don't you wish you could fly? You can, if only in your mind's eye. Stand upright, take three deep cleansing breaths, doing your belly breathing. Bend over at the waist. Extend your arms out. Shut your eyes and see yourself as a beautiful baby bird at the edge of the Grand Canyon with the other side a mile across. You want to soar. When you are ready, step off the edge, flap your wings and FLY! You can make it to the other side. We never know if we'll be successful until we try. You are a bird. Birds fly. Yes, sometimes even eagles need a push. Take a chance. Feel the exhilaration of doing something new, something scary. Dare to fly.

10. DICTION

We need to speak distinctly. Clench a pencil in your teeth and try reading the newspaper. Pronounce each syllable and word. Listen to your errors. Pronunciation is essential for all successes. Distinguish between the tongue and the lips that may be causing your diction challenges.

11. SOUND YOGA

Inhale through your nose and while you are exhaling chant each letter of the alphabet. Chant one letter until all the air is out of your lungs before going on to the next letter. Change the tone and pitch of your voice. Pay attention to the resonance of the sounds you are making.

12. NO IS A COMPLETE SENTENCE

Stand straight, rib cage up, shoulders back, good posture position. Say firmly and energetically three times "NO". Use your eyes, your body, your powerful being to express yourself. Try it in different voices. Know "NO".

13. PUPPET ON A STRING

Stand up straight. Take a deep breath and pull an imaginary string from the top of your head towards the stars. As you exhale, bring your arm down, shoulders rotate back. Take another breath. Look at yourself in the mirror and see yourself standing in a power stance.

14. BELLY LAUGH

Grab your stomach and laugh, laugh, laugh, until your laughter is real and unforced. Your cares will melt away. Laughing is terrific therapy for those days when you just can't get going. Get your endorphins pumped—laugh!

15. SMILEMAKER

When you are feeling low, put a smile on your face. It may be forced at first, but it is impossible to frown when you are smiling. Walk down the street and smile at everyone you see. Be genuine. In no time flat, you will be feeling happy as your smile will have made others smile also.

16. EYES AND MOUTH

Open your eyes as wide as you possibly can. Now squint your eyes until they are almost shut but you can still see. Quickly do both in reverse order. Open your mouth wide, wider, widest until you can't stretch it anymore. Now pucker up into the smallest mouth ever. Pair together a big mouth with big eyes, little mouth with little eyes. Then switch off, big mouth, little eyes, now try little mouth with big eyes. Do at least three different versions.

17. ICE CREAM TONGUE

Sweep your tongue around your lips as if you are licking up the tastiest ice cream ever. Stick your tongue out as far as it can go, curl it, do tongue tricks. Loosen up your mouth before attempting to negotiate any deal or audition for that big part!

18. IMAGINE

Children are great at imagining they are whoever they want to be. Become a child for awhile, find a room that has a full length mirror. Go inside, lock the door, look in the mirror and become the person you want to be most. Be the rock star, the pro ball player, Miss America, an astronaut, the President, win your Academy Award, a Purple heart, or the love of your life. Sing, dance, applaud, scream, yodel, travel to distant shores. Imagination is the beginning of reality. Savor the winning moment.

19. TONGUE TWISTERS

There's nothing better to get your mouth into shape that tongue twisters. Begin by saying each one slowly and distinctly. Increase speed as you feel confident. Every time a mistake is made, go back to the beginning and start again slowly. Your goal is to go as fast as you can. Whenever you feel tongue tied, whether it be at work, play, school, or family situation, take a few seconds to run through a couple of tongue twisters. They are a real ice-breaker. You'll usually get others to try them as well. Soon everyone will be giggling.
Here are a few of my favorites:

1. How many cuckoos could a good cook cook if a good cook could cook cuckoos?

2. Sicky licked sixty sticky stickers.

3. Tom tried to trap ten terrible tigers.

4. Bring that black book back.

5. Bobby broke Barry's baby bottle.

6. Betty Biddle's batter bakes better biscuits

7. The big black bug bit the big black bear and the big black bear began to bleed.

8. Six, slippery, slimy snakes sleep soundly.

9. She sells sea shells by the seashore.

10. Trudy tried to twist tough taffy Tuesday.

11. Candy can't can creamy carrots 'cause Candy can't can.

12. Round the rugged rock the ragged rascal ran.

13. Which wrist watch is a Swiss wrist watch.

14. He sits in her slip and sips Schlitz.

15. Peter Piper picked a peck of pickled peppers. How many pickled peppers did Peter Piper pick?

16. I'm a sheet slitter, I slit sheets. I'm the best sheet slitter that ever slit a sheet.

17. Pool players paradise produces playful products.

20. HOW GREAT I AM

This exercise requires keeping a journal or notebook. It can be as simple or fancy as you wish. When ever anyone gives you a compliment, no matter how small, the compliment gets written in your "How Great I Am" journal. **RULE ONE: ABSOLUTELY NO NEGATIVES IN HERE, NO BUTS, SHOULDS, ETC.** For example, someone may say: "your hair looks very pretty today." You write: "I have pretty hair." If someone says, "you wrote the proposal well but you had several typos." You write: "I am a good writer." Please note, the "but" and criticism are not part of this exercise no matter how well meant or helpful. This book is ONLY for great things. At the end of each day, before retiring to sleep, read "How great I am" and your dreams will be filled with greatness. Before long, you will believe in yourself and the possibilities of your greatness. Soon you will be saying a simple, "thank you" to compliments instead of always trying to explain what is wrong with you. You were born to be great. Don't make excuses for flaws. Be great.

21. I AM THE GREATEST!

This exercise is best done in a small group of either friends, family, or a classroom, however it can be done alone. Everyone joins hands and sends a positive squeeze around the group. (If alone hold your hands in a victory grasp) Take a deep breath, throw your arms in the air, pound your chest and yell, "I am the GREATEST!" Believe it and do it three times. This is so empowering.

22. COLOR MY WORLD

Whenever you are feeling extremely jubilant a wonderful way to record the experience is by doing a freeform drawing of you and the world you live in today. Use lots of colors, express, and have fun. Label this drawing with the date and occasion of your happiness and save in your "How Great I Am" journal. Whenever you are having a bad day, buy a new box of colored crayons in anticipation of feeling better!

23. BODY LANGUAGE

Our bodies express what our words do or don't say. Get familiar with how you communicate. If you have a video camera, set it up and position it to run automatically as you go through these exercises. If you don't have a camera, try this in front of your mirror. When using the mirror, make sure the actions your body makes replicates what the emotions or words are trying to say.

For example, act out the following:

☆ surprise ☆ pain ☆ joy ☆ hunger ☆ cold

☆ desperation ☆ confusion ☆ anger ☆ beauty

☆ frustration ☆ exhilaration ☆ serenity ☆ strenght

☆ exhaustion ☆ love ☆ admiration ☆ happiness

☆ compassion ☆ fear ☆ weakness ☆ nervousness

Our bodies do talk. Can you "see" what they are saying?

24. MOVEMENT WITHOUT WORDS

This time, try moving your body without using your voice. Think a sentence in your head and then watch what your body does. Are your body movements indicative of what you want to relay?

For example, how would you say "I don't know" ? Would you shrug your shoulders, perhaps? Try thinking the following and use your body to indicate the feelings:

☆ I love you ☆ Get away from me ☆ Be quiet

☆ I can do this myself ☆ I want that ☆ I'm scared

☆ Not again! ☆ Why me? ☆ Thank you ☆ I won

☆ This is fun ☆ Life is great ☆ That stinks

☆ Who, me? ☆ How beautiful! ☆ This is hard work

☆ I'm really tired ☆ I feel terrific ☆ Who's that?

25. TELL ME ABOUT YOURSELF

This is the number one asked question in the acting industry. However, when you think about it, it is probably the number one asked question in the world, regardless of the profession. Unfortunately, most of us answer by retorting: "What do you want to know?" Think about the question carefully. Who are you and what do you do that would inspire, interest, and motivate others to want to know more about you. Don't give a litany of awards, jobs, or accomplishments. Instead focus on three areas that are your passion and speak about them with intensity, focus, and clarity. Don't ramble. Be succinct. Tape record your voice. Listen for inflection, excitement, and determination.

Do you like you? Do you like what you are saying? Would you like to be your friend? If not, change your dialogue, adjust, correct, delete, and start again. Do this until you feel totally comfortable that the next time someone asks you to tell them about yourself you will engage them with your spontaneity and love of life.

26. NAME GAME

Try saying your name in a different voice. Try accents, various emotions, express yourself. Who is the real you?

27. MEAN MACHINE

Do you know what sounds machines make? Do machines have a language? Make a list of all the machines you can think of. Now use your imagination and try imitating the machine in both movement and sound. Aren't you glad you are human?

28. BALLOONS

When you are over stressed, try being a balloon. Let your feelings blow you up until you can't get any bigger. Then go ahead and pop, plopping on the floor in a heap. Repeat this exercise several times until you are feeling relived of the tension.

29. FAIRY GODMOTHER

Imagine that you are a fairy godmother/godfather who has a magic wand. You can even make a magic wand from a stick, add a few ribbons, and presto, you hold the key to the kingdom. Wave the magic wand over your head when you need an additional boost. Remember that you hold the magic to create the life you want inside yourself. Dream it, do it.

30. MAGAZINE MAGIC

Cut photos and sayings out of magazines that embody the person you know that is captive inside. Create a collage of any size. Add to it whenever the desire hits. I find it helpful to put this creation in my "How Great I Am" journal. Be positive, realistic, and hopeful. Take the actions required to BE the you that is.

31. MY ACCOMPLISHMENTS

Write down all the things you know how to do, (besides acting) or do routinely. Don't leave anything out, no matter how mundane you may feel it is. For example, "I can repair PVC pipes, plant a garden, take out the garbage, paint a wall, read to children, wash dishes, vacuum the rug, drive a car, write a letter, type on the computer, program a VCR..." See how smart you already are!

32. BUTTERFLIES

Have an imaginary butterfly land on your open palm. Admire the beauty, the fine details of the wings. Stand quietly and see this magnificent creature. Now place the imaginary butterfly on an imaginary plant and feel the exhilaration of letting go.

33. THE TELEPHONE

The telephone rings. Answer it knowing that the person on the other line has the potential to offer you the career you have been dreaming of for years. How do you respond? Have a normal conversation. Be enthusiastic. Be prepared to answer questions. Be prepared to ask questions. Be prepared...period. It is helpful to refer to the exercise "Tell me about yourself" (number 25) and also to tape record this possible future conversation for a future audition.

34. THE GIFT

When you walk into a room, what are your first sensations? Are you afraid you may not be wanted, that your zipper is down, that you are not good enough, or any number of other negative thoughts. STOP, LOOK, LISTEN! You are a gift. Regard everyone you meet as a gift to you and you as a gift to them. Believe people are waiting to make a deal with you. They want and need you in their life. Once you believe this, your body language will convey THE GIFT OF YOU.

THE FOLLOWING FIVE EXERCISES (#35 -#39) ARE IMPROVISATIONAL GAMES THAT WORK BETTER WITH THREE OR MORE INDIVIDUALS. THESE ARE PERFECT FOR A FAMILY, A GROUP OF FRIENDS, OR A WORKSHOP.

35. ONE WORD STORY

At least three people sit together. If more than three people are in the group, it is best to sit in a circle. Each person gets to say only one word. The purpose is to create a story by using LISTENING skills. Most stories end up having a humorous appeal which works wonders for the soul. The story always begins with "Once upon a time, there was....". Have fun and say the first word that comes to your mind. This exercise can quickly have everyone in the room laughing. Listening is the key to success.

36. MIRROR, MIRROR

How good are you at mirroring other people's actions, emotions, and body language? This exercise requires two people facing one another. One person is designated as the actor, the other is the mirror. The mirror must follow exactly the actions of the actor. After a time, switch places. What we can learn is to mirror others in conversation. People tend to like those who are most like themselves. Therefore in awkward or stressful situations, if we model the behavior of our opponent in voice inflection, body language, and tonality we tend to do better.

37. ACTOR REACTOR

All acting is reacting. For any action there is an immediate reaction, whether good or bad. Similar to Mirror, Mirror, in this exercise one person is the ACTOR; the other is the REACTOR. Whatever the ACTOR does, the

REACTOR must portray a realistic reaction to the action. Learn from your colleague what response your actions take. Is it what you expected? This is a very powerful exercise to help you see yourself as others see you. Be honest and don't try to be funny.

38. NOISES

Everyone in the group shuts their eyes. One person makes a noise, the person sitting to the right tries to imitate it, the person sitting next to the right imitates the former... and around the circle the noise goes until the noise is no longer the same noise.

39. MECHANICAL CONCERT

Using different inanimate objects, like a chair, a spoon, and a shoe, three people try to make sounds by pushing, pounding, pinging, grinding whatever object they have chosen to make music as a group concert. Requires listening and cooperation.

40. POWER OF THE BRAIN

The brain does not hear negatives, therefore it is very important how we phrase what we say. For example, if I said to my son: "Don't swing on the counter because you will fall and break your teeth", the only thing his brain will hear is "Swing on the counter, because you will fall and break your teeth." We need to find different ways of getting things done without using negatives. "I will not get sick" transfers to "I will get sick" so why not say "I choose to be healthy". Write down different ways you can reprogram the way you speak so that what you say is a positive statement instead of a negative instruction. Be aware of what you are telling your brain and the brains of others. Don't feel your big toe! (What are you feeling right now...I bet it is your big toe!)

41. SUCCESS DRESS

How you attire yourself says volumes about who you are at that moment in time. When I'm in the garden, I look like a gardener, complete with boots, old clothes, muddy gloves, floppy hat and all my tools. Strangers passing by my yard while I am working in it have told me that my employer works me too hard, not knowing that I am the employer. No one would mistake me for a beauty queen. I feel like a gardener, smell like a gardener, and act like a gardener. The fact is, I am a gardener when I am gardening. The same goes for other parts of life. If you want a certain part or job, dress for the role. It is said that life is not a dress rehearsal, so my suggestion is to wardrobe yourself for the success you want to achieve. If you are asked to audition for the part of a bank president, make sure you are wearing a well made tailored suit. If you are supposed to be a golfer, dress in golfing attire. Costuming ourselves actually helps get into character. A book is judged by its cover so make sure yours is what is expected. Look the part and the part is often yours.

42. THE TURTLE

Get on the ground in a turtle position. Try walking like a turtle. Stick your neck out. Look around. Now roll over on your back. Can you move? What do you see? Where do you feel more powerful, on your back or on your feet? Take measured risks, whenever you get turned upside down, remember to roll over.

43. ROCK OUT

There is nothing better for the soul than shaking your body and dancing around like a wild person. Turn the music on, dance to the beat, allow every part of your body to move to the music. Become the music. Let loose, be free, you are free!

44. SING A SONG

Next to rocking out, singing at the top of your lungs feels like heaven. Get in your car, roll up the windows, and SING. Who cares what your voice is like? Have fun and be part of the song. If you are at home, combine singing with dancing for the greatest work-out and energy booster around. Guaranteed to put a smile on your face.

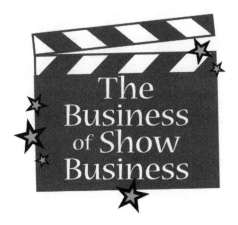

Chapter 23

Children and Acting...Laws, Information and Help

*"What gifts can we give our children?
Attention, for one day it will be too late.
A sense of value, the inalienable place of the
individual in the scheme of things, with all that
accrues to the individual self-reliance, courage,
conviction, self-respect, and respect for others.
A sense of humor. Laughter encourages life.
The meaning of discipline. If we falter at
discipline, life will do it for us.*

*The will to work. Satisfying work is
a lasting joy.
The talent for sharing, for it is not so much
what we give as what we share.
The love of justice. Justice is the bulwark
against violence and oppression and the
repository of human dignity.
The passion for truth, for truth is the
beginning of every good thing.
The power of faith which is a beacon of hope
lighting all darkness.
The knowledge of being loved beyond demand
or reciprocity, praise or blame, for those
so loved are never lost.
What shall we give our children?
Long days to be merry and nights without
fear...the memory of a good, loving home."*

Creative Dramatics for Children

Creative dramatics is concerned with the process of encouraging children to create informal drama through effective leadership. Drama is an art which nurtures creativity and sensibilities. A good play is always a story about what happens within the heart and mind of a person. In a good story, the protagonist is always in some kind of trouble. He becomes the person involved in a situation which motivates inner conflicts between the forces of good and evil. The audience identifies and feels with the protagonist as he struggles with these conflicting forces and eventually triumphs or yields to defeat. But, in the end, because of his moral convictions and actions, he always becomes a more admirable person. Then the audience identifies, they participate in the struggles. They meditate on the thoughts, feelings, and actions of mankind. Theatre is the central artistic symbol of the struggle between good and evil within men.

Good drama feeds a child's heart and mind and thus causes him to dwell in the realms of wonder. Entertainment is foremost in children's theatre, but itself fulfills certain psychological and developmental needs of young growing personalities. These needs have been expressed in various ways, such as:

1. The desire to see the abstract pleasure of pictures in imagination realized in a concrete form.
2. The craving for a conception of life higher than what the actual world offers.
3. The propensity to express the larger than life race of the individual.
4. An outlet for the natural drives for adventure and excitement.
5. The need to experience emotions that might not be evoked in everyday living.
6. The need to enter worlds larger than their own and there encounter people and adventures different from themselves.
7. The imaginative satisfaction for the ego and mutuality needs of the growing child.
8. The need to escape from inferiority, rid themselves of handicaps, compensate for weaknesses, fulfill thwarted desires and enjoy pleasure and desire.

Drama helps unlock inarticulate children. The desire to create is universal and the desire to dramatize is a basic human interest. No observers are allowed in my classroom to enable the child to free his creativity with an undivided heart and mind in a non-judgmental environment. Feelings are allowed and encouraged and everyone is accepted for who he is as an individual.

Teaching is a labor of love. A great teacher must have a PLUS quality....energy, compassion, humor, imagination, perception, humility, patience, wisdom, taste, judgment, joy, sorrow, big shoulders and listening ears. Teachers must motivate with kindness and enthusiasm enabling children to discover, encourage, endure, enjoy, guide, create, and dramatize. When children are inspired they will have fun, leaving each class and learning situation with a greater sense of discovery of their inner being, increased self-esteem and personal power.

Producers, directors, and casting agents are looking for natural, energetic, yet well-behaved children. Children need to display a sense of security and a willingness to work without their parents around. Children should not be robotic, should have talent and be good readers and interpreters of dialog. They need to be comfortable in front of a camera, alone in a room, part of a large crowd. They must act mature and friendly. Impromptu spontaneity is important. They can not act programmed or rehearsed. NATURAL is key. Kids need to be able to think on their feet, be easy going, have discipline, a sense of self-esteem and confidence in their ability. They have to be willing to work with strangers and in some uncomfortable locations. Often other adults "strangers" will be playing their parents and other kids may play the role of siblings. Adaptability is essential. It is important that they are not "know it all's" and can take direction. Outgoing, great personality, verbal, good speakers are qualities that all the agents are asking for.

Appearance

Again, natural, normal kids are in. Real kids, straight from the playgrounds...not over-dressed or over-groomed.

For girls, unless specified, no bows in the hair, no fancy ribbons, no jewelry. Boys and girls should not wear clothing with logos on them. Bright colors are best and clean school clothes are almost always appropriate. Watch commercials and magazine ads for the latest look. Look clean, but like a kid.

Character kids, ethnic and Asian boys are the most needed group at this writing. Boys are usually in more demand than girls in all ethnicity and age ranges.

Parents

Overbearing stage parents are the thorn in the side of directors, agents and producers. Clients are actually asking not to see certain children because they can't stand the parents. As a stage mom or dad it is best to be supportive, but in the background. (Think...fly on the wall) Remember it is the child who is auditioning or acting, not you. Let the child's acting technique speak for itself.

Products

Most children's commercial calls are for toys, food, video games, or as part of a family outing. Get as much information from your agent about the product as possible. If the product is Coca Cola, go drink the soft drink so you know what it tastes like . Get familiar with the product you may be working with., When you work on your script, you will have a more effective emotional recall and remember the taste.

Finding a Coach

One of the most important steps you can take in improving your child's chances for success in acting is to find a good coach. A coach needs to be a motivator, some one active in the industry, and someone the child can look up to, respect, and emulate. It is exciting for kids when a teacher is busy doing commercials, TV shows, and stage productions as this brings fresh ideas and techniques to the child. A coach who is "out there" auditioning has more understanding of the rejection, the nervousness and the fear that all is part of the process. A good coach will set small reachable tasks and not let fear rule. A good coach not only inspires but listens. A good coach encourages the child to act like a child, not like a small adult. Auditions are fun when the child is prepared. Remember that a coach cannot guarantee a job...no one can do that, but the odds are better of your child getting work when he/she knows what to expect. Probably only about 20 children in American earn $250,000 a year or more, so don't go into this business thinking that your child will make your family independently wealthy. Trust your coach to keep you balanced.

Do's and Don'ts for Parents

It's not easy being a parent of an actor. Every parent thinks that "my child" is the most talented, gorgeous, bookable kid in the world. This fabulous child of yours is going to be rejected more often than not. This is show business and everybody wants a part of it. For you, the parent, much dedication and hard work are involved. You are required to drive the child to auditions and jobs at very unreasonable times. You or an authorized guardian must stay with your child on the set at all times. And, you, the parent, are not often given much respect. Also, you are never paid for your time or expenses. It is a thankless job being the parent of a working child actor or model. Producers and directors wish they did not have to deal with parents at all, but until a child is 18, the law states that parents must accompany the child. So, you can either be a "good" stage parent or a "bad" stage parent. Here are tips to help you help your child:

☆ Let your child fulfill his/her dreams. Don't assume acting is their dream because it is yours.

☆ Make sure your child is ready for auditions by having had enough sleep, food, and schoolwork completed.

☆ Don't be pushy, let your child be seen and heard, not you.

☆ Be prepared to do a lot of chauffeuring for auditions, callbacks, and jobs. Be ready for anything.

☆ Don't pay money for expensive photographs, modeling classes, or representation. Get a reliable, trustworthy coach first.

☆ Explain to your child what is going to happen and that he/she may not get the job, but the most important thing is to have fun and enjoy.

☆ This is an opportunity for your child to grow as a person, show your child that you care by listening.

☆ Let your child lead a balanced life outside of acting with friends, school activities, extracurricular sports, or just plain kid pursuits.

☆ Don't bank on your child supporting you.

☆ Be always vigilant on your child's behalf, but keep a respectful and watchful distance.

☆ If after a time, your child decides to take a break, let it be OK.

☆ Have confidence in your child that he/she will succeed in whatever life choices are made.

☆ Keep work permits current...there is nothing more disheartening to a child than getting booked on a job and not being able to accept it because mom or dad did not renew the work permit.

☆ Make sure your child keeps up with schoolwork.

☆ Always have your child's interest at heart, don't sign any contract that doesn't feel right. If an agent wants your child today, your child will be wanted tomorrow. Don't rush into anything.

More than anything, love your child because your child is a good human being. When your child's acting career comes to a halt, you need to be there to offer support. Don't let Hollywood determine the life of your child. The positive side of acting is increased self-confidence and self-direction, meeting exciting famous people, traveling to exotic locations, financial rewards, great food and lots of fun. Young performers, if not guided correctly, can pay a high personal price. National standards in education, transportation, work hours, supervision, interviews, medical care, and meals are still in the process of being developed and adopted. There is a parent trap...stay out of it!

Most Often Asked Questions for Minors

1. What is the age definition of a minor under their major Union contracts?

For commercials	14 & under
Film/TV	Under 18
Industrials	Under 18
Network Code	14 & under
Public Radio	"School-age"
Radio Commercial	"School-age"
Radio Programming	"School-age"
Public TV	Under 15

2. What are the total hours a minor may be allowed to actually work?
Film/TV/Network Code on school days

Under 6=	3 hours
age 6-8 =	4 hours
age 9-15=	5 hours
age 16-17=	6 hours

3. What are the daily school time requirements for a minor?

Film/TV/Network Code

Under 6=	0 hours
age 6-17=	3 hours

4. During what hours do the contracts allow interviews?

Most codes are after school and before 8pm. Film/TV allows interviews until 9pm. Print work interviews and go-see's happen at all hours.

5. When do the provisions for minors in the Union Contract take precedence over state law?

Only when state provisions are LESS RESTRICTIVE than the contract provision.

6. May I watch my child while he/she is working?

Yes! You ALWAYS have the right to be within sight and sound of your child, except when space does not permit (small sets or crowded control rooms, for example); in such instances, you may be as close as feasible. During auditions, for the most part, parents are not allowed in the room. Always be a "fly on the wall" and keep out of the way. If you have a concern for your child at any time, talk to the set teacher or the assistant director only.

7. What kind of identification is necessary on a set?

Always bring your child's social security card, your child's union membership cards, a valid work permit, your child's passport or birth certificate, and your own driver's license as proof of parentage.

8. What other items should I bring?

Tissues, wash cloth, snacks, books, toys, games, water, any special foods or medication which you require, warm clothing, rain gear, school books and assignments.

9. Will my child be paid for supplying wardrobe?

In most cases, yes, your child is entitled to reimbursement for wearing his/her own clothing while performing.

10. To whom do we report when we arrive on the set?

Find the Stage Manager or the Assistant Director. They should direct you to the person responsible for dealing with your child. You should also report to the set teacher, if one is present.

11. Will a dressing room be provided for my child?

Yes, and your child may not share it with an adult or a minor of the opposite sex. This is the law!

12. May I bring other children, a friend or a relative to the set where my child is working?

NO! NO! NO! Leave your friends, other children, your pets, and relatives at home. The professional method to follow is: one parent for one child.

13. What if I am unable to personally accompany my child to the set?

There must always be an adult present for each child. If the parent can't attend, a guardian must be appointed and a legal guardianship form filled out to be given to the set teacher or AD. (A sample is included in this book)

14. What if I must leave the set while my child is working?

Another adult must be appointed as the child's guardian with a written authorization for medical attention. (See the sample guardianship form in this book)

15. Will my child have to do stunts?

Any hazardous activity can be refused. Most stunts are determined on an individual basis and must utilize a stunt contract in addition to your regular contract.

16. Does the production company make a check out to me?

No, your child is the person working and your child will be paid. Most states have adopted legislation which requires the parent to set up a blocked trust fund for the minor to protect the child's assets. In California this law is called "The Coogan Law" named after the child actor Jackie Coogan. Some production companies will not employ your child until proof of this trust fund has been shown.

17. Are children eligible for unemployment benefits?

In most states minors do qualify for unemployment compensation. Your child has worked, the employer has paid the assessment, and the child is legally entitled.

18. What is emancipation and is it a good idea?

Emancipation is a court order declaring a child to be a legal adult. People opt for this action in order to work as an adult. Check with your state about the provisions and benefits.

19. When I accompany my child on location, who pays my expenses?

Agents negotiate the specifics of the child's contract which need to include provisions for the parent. In general, the Producer pays for accommodations, transportation and meals on location. There is no salary for the parent, however, unless negotiated.

California Child Labor Laws for The Entertainment Industry

"Each child brings his own blessing into the world."

Yiddish Proverb

All children under the age of 18 must have a valid entertainment work permit. The age definition of a minor under a major union contract is any performer 17 years of age or younger. Exceptions to this rule apply only to performers who have already satisfied compulsory state education requirements, or are married, members of the armed forces or legally emancipated. Various state regulations apply, so check your particular state laws for specifics. Labor code #1308.5 requires the written consent of the Labor Commissioner for any minor to be employed in the modeling, theatrical or entertainment industry. Any person, agent, parent or guardian who employs or permits any minor to be employed in violation of this section is guilty of a misdemeanor. You may obtain a copy of the entertainment work permit application from the Department of Industrial Relations, division of Labor Standards and Enforcement in your state. It may be copied, filled out and presented in person or by mail to the Department of Industrial Relations, division of Labor Standards and Enforcement for a permit. Requirements are as follows:

☆ If child is under school age, a parent need only complete and sign the front of the application and provide the labor commissioner's office with a copy of the child's birth certificate or passport as proof of age.

☆ If the child is of school age, a parent must complete and sign the front of the application. A certified school official (including teacher, principal, vice-principal, or counselor) must sign and complete the school record portion of the back acknowledging and specifying that the minor's health, attendance, and school grades are all satisfactory or better. If the school authority is not available during a school break or vacation, a parent can provide the original of the child's latest report card in lieu of the school signature and proof of age. A doctor's signature for health is required.

Entertainment permits are valid for six months and renewable by mail, but do allow 2-6 weeks before the needed date.

I advise obtaining the first application by visiting in person, then renew by mail afterwards. Bring the completed forms to these locations, or check your yellow pages for the location nearest you in your city or state.

Northern California locations can be reached at 415-557-7878 for a recorded message.

☆ SAN FRANCISCO: 30 Van Ness Street, 3rd floor

☆ OAKLAND: 1515 Clay Street #801

☆ SAN JOSE: 100 Paseo de San Antonio, # 120

☆ SACRAMENTO: 2422 Arden Way, #50

☆ SANTA ROSA: 50 "d" Street, #360

☆ STOCKTON: 31 East Channel Street #328

Sumary of Work Hours

Age 15 days to 6 months:

☆ Two hours of maximum time on set with hours between 9:30am & 11:30am or between 2:30pm & 4:30pm only, with 20 minutes of work activity.

☆ One studio teacher and one nurse must be present for each 3 or fewer infants 15 days to 6 weeks old. One studio teacher and one nurse must be present for each 10 or fewer infants 6 weeks to 6 months old.

Six months to 2 years:

☆ Two hours work activity, 4 hours maximum time on set, balance for rest and recreation.

☆ One studio teacher required for 10 minors, one per 20 on weekend and vacations.

☆ Minors may be tutored between the hours of 8am & 4pm.

Two years to 6 years:

☆ Three hours work activity, 6 hours maximum time on set, balance for rest and recreation. May only work between 5am & 12:30am.

☆ One studio teacher required for 10 minors, one per 20 on weekend and vacations.

☆ Minors may be tutored between the hours of 8am & 4pm.

Six years to 9 years:

☆ When school is in session, child may work 4 hours, 3 hours of schooling, 1 hour rest and recreation with a maximum of 8 hours on set.

☆ On non-work days, child may work 6 hours, with 1 hour of rest and recreation and a 7 hour workday maximum

☆ All work may occur only between 5 am and 12:30am (10pm preceding school days more than 4 hours long.

☆ One studio teacher required for 10 minors, one per 20 on weekend and vacations.

☆ Minors may be tutored between the hours of 8am & 4pm.

Nine years to 16 years:

☆ When school is in session, child may work for 5 hours, with 3 hours of schooling, 1 hour of rest and recreation for a total of 9 hours on the set.

☆ On non-work days, child may work for 7 hours with 1 hour rest and recreation for a total of 8 hours on set.

☆ All work may occur only between 5 am and 12:30am (10pm preceding school days more than 4 hours long.

☆ One studio teacher required for 10 minors, one per 20 on weekend and vacations.

☆ Minors may be tutored between the hours of 8am & 4pm.

Sixteen years to 18 years:

☆ When school is in session, child may work for 6 hours, with 3 hours of schooling, 1 hour of rest and recreation for a total of 10 hours on the set.

☆ On non-work days, child may work for 7 hours with 1 hour rest and recreation for a total of 8 hours on set.

☆ All work may occur only between 5 am and 12:30 am (10 pm preceding school days more than 4 hours long.

☆ Studio teacher required only for minors' schooling, if minor still required to attend school.

General notes:

☆ No minor may work over 8 hours in a day (Labor Code #1308.7, 1392) or over 48 hours in a week. No exceptions.

☆ Meal periods are not work time. Workday may only be extended up to one-half hour for a meal period. (8 CCR 11761) Meals must be within 6 hours of call time and/or previous meal period. Studio teachers may require an earlier meal period.

☆ Travel between studio and location is work time.

The Coogan Law-protecting minors money

Most people have heard of the famous child actor Jackie Coogan. What many may not know is that in the 1930's he sued his parents to recover the $4 million he had earned as a child star that they had squandered. The collection of his fortune proved to be in vain because in those days a child's earnings was the property of the parents. Therefore when Jackie entered adulthood he discovered that he was penniless along with many other child actors whose parents had not protected their assets. California enacted a law in 1939 named after the actor to ensure that child actors received a portion of the earnings they amassed while they were working in the entertainment field as minors.

In the year 2000, the New Coogan Law protecting young performers earnings went into effect. This new law covers every job performed by child actors, sports figures and musicians, including all commercials, movies, TV shows, stage plays, concerts, print work and background work-basically any work that a child does for pay in the entertainment, music and sports worlds.

The new changes do the following:

☆ cover 100% of all minors' contracts, whether court-approved or not;

☆ require that 15% of a child's gross earnings be placed in a trust account for the minor until the age of 18. (The remaining 85% can be used for payment of operating expenses such as commissions to agents and managers, attorney and accounting fees, acting coaching, professional photographs, transportation costs, advertisement and other necessary acting expenses);

☆ make the earnings the separate property of the child, not the community property of the parent;

☆ require producers to make deposits within 15 business days directly into the trust account so that interest may accrue immediately on the principal earnings.

Setting up a Coogan Account is easy. Just walk into a bank, brokerage firm, credit union, or savings and loan within seven days of signing a contract and ask to set up a "Coogan Account". Forms will be given to you specifically for this New Coogan Law. If for any reason your financial institution has not heard of these forms, have them contact SAG at 323-549-6663 or 212-944-1030 immediately to obtain forms. You can also email: govrelat@sag.org. The trust can be set up anywhere in or outside the United States. Although it is a California law, if the production company is based in California, the minor must have this special trust account. If a producer fails to comply with the 15th business day/15% deposit, please contact SAG to help you with compliance.

It is important that all parents and guardians understand their responsibilities as fiduciary trustees under the amended law. Again, if a parent has questions, Screen Actors Guild is available to answer. You can also consult legal counsel or a financial advisor. This new law is in the best interests of our child actors and protects them from unscrupulous activities by parents and guardians. Hopefully our child entertainers will be able to finance a college education, purchase a home, and provide for themselves and their family with the money earned as young performers because of the enforcement of this important new law.

Emancipated Minors

Child performers can earn millions of dollars in the entertainment field. There is much confusion on whether an emancipated child is exempt from education on the set. An emancipated minor can manage his or her own financial matters, receive a work permit, get medical attention and enter into contract negotiations all without the consent of a parent or a guardian. However, emancipation does not necessarily exempt the minor from the child labor laws and regulations of the state, including compulsory school attendance. An emancipated minor may not work longer hours than a non-emancipated child. If the child is under eighteen years of age and has not graduated from high school or obtained a high school proficiency certificate (which is available to only 16 and 17 year olds,) the minor must be provided a minimum of three hours of education on the set. In California, a studio teacher must be available on all sets where minors are working for both educational and safety purposes. As with all minors, the New Coogan Law applies to emancipated children. The laws in California have implications in other states as well, so always check the laws of your state before accepting production work.

Legal Guardianship Form

This form must be filled out by the parent or legal guardian when entrusting another person as a legal guardian for your child. The appointed guardian is to be present at all times with the child during filming.

I,_____, parent or legal guardian of_____, have entrusted my child into the care of,_____,an adult, for the particular reasons for a temporary period of time and for the welfare of the child.

In such connection I authorize said caring adult to consent to any X-ray examination, anesthetic, medical, dental, or surgical diagnosis or treatment or hospital care, to be rendered to said minor under the general or special supervision, and on the advice of a physician and/or surgeon and/or dentist licensed under the provisions of the Medical Practice Act.

Whenever_____ consents to such medical and/or surgical and/or dental care, it shall be as if I myself had considered and consented to it.

Signed:_____

Relationship to Minor:_____

Date:_____

Time Period:_____

Printed name:_____

Address:_____

Personal Physician:_____

Insurance information:_____

Other Telephone numbers:_____

Any special notes:_____

Special Information

PARENTS AND GUARDIANS: A parent or guardian over 21 years of age must accompany a minor under 16 years of age on all sets and locations. The rule applies to wardrobe, make-up, hairstyling, and audio recording as well as acting on the set. A guardian must possess written authorization from the parent for medical emergencies.

STUDIO TEACHERS: A studio teacher is required by California state law to be present on every set where a child is working. There are over 300 studio teachers in the state of California. Your child has the RIGHT to a teacher on the set. This includes photography, recording, modeling, theatrical productions, feature films, TV shows, commercials, and any other performance where minors perform to entertain the public. In addition to teaching, the studio teacher has the responsibility for caring for the health, safety, and morals of minors. If the parent is uncomfortable with any situation involving the child, the studio teacher is the person to address the concern. The child will receive an EXCUSED ABSENCE from school if a studio teacher is present. Do not accept an unexcused absence. The schools are entitled to all state money including the average daily attendance money for all students working with a set teacher. If the school has any questions, please have them contact the Labor Commission for clarification.

"Each day of our lives, we make deposits in the memory banks of our children."

Charles Swindoll

Chapter 24

Ready, Set, Action...What to Expect Once You are Cast!

"The harder I work, the luckier I get"
James Thurber

The telephone rings and your agent exclaims: "You got the job!" These are the words actors live to hear. You are excited, overwhelmed, thrilled. Now what? Follow these simple guidelines.

Questions to ask your agent:
   ☆ Time of call
   ☆ Name of production company, report to contact name
   ☆ Address of location

☆ wardrobe requirements

☆ contract or pay scale you will be working under

Your responsibilities:

☆ Confirm with your agent or casting director

☆ Get good maps and find the location (do not ask directions)

☆ Prepare your wardrobe, including ironing. Don't forget shoes, socks, stockings, and accessories to match. It is always a good idea to bring 3 or 4 changes of wardrobe "just in case." (For extra work, always bring extra wardrobe as each change you actually wear will be financially compensated)

☆ If asked to come 'camera ready' (which is usual for extra work), come with make-up and hair complete.

☆ Bring a book or work to do during down time.

☆ If a minor, bring your work permit and a parent or legal guardian who will stay with you all day. No extra persons allowed.

☆ If over 18, come alone.

☆ Bring documents for I-9's including drivers license or birth certificate and social security card, or passport.

☆ Bring a pen and daytimer or electronic organizer

☆ If you get sick or lost the day of the shoot, contact your agent first or the casting person who booked you for assistance.

☆ Know your lines.

☆ Be on time.

When you get to the set:

☆ Check in with the AD or whoever is in charge.

☆ Go to wardrobe or make-up if necessary.

☆ Stay in the area where you are told to congregate and keep quiet. Get prepared for the shoot. Never leave the set for any reason without permission.

☆ Listen for directions.

☆ Be prepared for a long day.

☆ Make sure to return all items to the production company that they provided for your use.

☆ Use of drugs or alcohol is prohibited.

☆ Do not ask for photographs or autographs unless you are a principal character and have a good working relationship with the person to whom you are requesting a photo or autograph. For extra players, this behavior is prohibited.

☆ Say thank you and follow up with a thank you note.

When you work you are representing the agent or casting service that booked you. Always be professional, courteous, and prompt. For any disagreements or problems, contact your agent immediately.

Checklist of What to Bring on a Job or Audition or Just Keep in Your Car

Keep the following items in your car in a duffel bag so that you are always ready for an audition:

☆ maps

☆ comb/brush

☆ hairspray

☆ toothbrush/toothpaste

☆ washcloth/wipes

☆ water bottle

☆ body lotion/cream

☆ lip gloss/sunscreen

☆ snacks

☆ books/toys
☆ homework for kids
☆ change of clothes
☆ warm jacket
☆ pillow and blanket
☆ umbrella
☆ portfolio/head shot/resume/business cards
☆ weekly calendar, day timer, and phone directory
☆ required documents: Driver's license, social security card,
☆ passport or birth certificate, vouchers, contracts, work permits, doctors letter of immunizations (kids only)
☆ Change of clothing (shorts, tennis shoes, t-shirt, casual dress, long pants)
☆ Plenty of quarters for parking meters

It's always better to be prepared

Chapter 25

Extra Work

"I am somebody. I am me. I like being me. And I need nobody to make me somebody."
Louis L'Amour

Extra work, also referred to as background work, is an important part of any TV or film project. Although most people aspire to being principal actors, extra work is an avenue to scope out the possibilities and get familiar with the film and television business. I am a big proponent of "actors acting" which translates that we actors need to focus our outside jobs on working in this business. For example, why is it when you travel to Los Angeles every waiter you meet is really an "actor." I say "this is a waiter waiting to be an actor." Actors act and if that means taking extra jobs to pay the bills and get experience, go for it. Extra work provides an excellent opportunity to meet people in the industry and to get on the job experience. Extra work is an avenue for those new to the business or a new area who are seeking acting employment. Background work for film and TV does not pay much more than minimum wage but is great compensation for commercials. There are people, including agents, who will advise aspiring actors to shy away from extra work because of being labeled an extra. As long as you don't list extra work inappropriately on your resume and you are up front in interview situations regarding your work as an extra, I feel you will benefit from the experience. You may even get lucky and get upgraded to a principal which several of my clients and colleagues have over the years.

If you greatly dislike doing extra work or your agent is vehemently opposed, don't do it. Never take an extra job over a principal audition. Trust your instinct on how much background work you want to do. Sometimes being an extra on a film is the only route you may have of working with a director or star whose work you greatly admire. Would you rather have the opportunity to work on the set, or sit home and wish you were working? For example, my clients who have worked on projects where Robin Williams was acting felt that they had been paid to watch a fine performance by an Academy winning actor and comedian.

When you do decide to do extra work, here are some helpful hints:

    ☆ let all the local casting people know you are interested in doing background work by sending them 5 head shots, resumes, and a current snapshot for their background files.

☆ Register with casting companies for background work. Many have web sites that list union and non-union productions for which extras are needed. Use these sites.

☆ Check casting hotlines for upcoming work.

☆ Maintain a large wardrobe, including costumes and period pieces and make sure the casting people know you have this asset. Visit http://badfads.com for a collection of fashion trends from the past 100 years.

☆ You have cars or animals that may be appropriate for work, make sure they are on file with you.

☆ When called for jobs, be enthusiastic and upbeat, take the info and then SHOW UP ON TIME.

☆ Be easy to work with. If you are dependable, friendly, and professional, your chances of working with the same casting director are greatly increased.

☆ If you are not union, but interested in getting into the union, let the casting person know that you are available as a Taft-Hartley, if they need you.

☆ On the set, pay attention to the work, and the Assistant Director's (AD) directions. Don't complain with other performers.

☆ You may get lucky and be upgraded, so stay within sight and sound of the AD. Be enthusiastic, professional, and have fun. You are getting free training while you learn the business of show business.

☆ Extra work is not glamorous or financially rewarding but with enough experience you can definitely augment your career with inside knowledge while meeting interesting people. ENJOY the ride!

Upgrades

Many people do extra work in the hopes of being upgraded to a principal performer. Being upgraded happens more often than most people think and when it happens to you...well...congratulations, you've hit the jackpot! Under the Theatrical and Television contracts of SAG there are only two ways to be upgraded from background performer to principal performer:

1. Be directed to speak lines

2. Perform a stunt

Commercials, however, offer the extra two additional avenues to be upgraded to principal.

3. Be alone on screen, photographed by a stationary camera and is identified with the product or service.

4. Be identifiable, in the foreground, and illustrates a product or service or illustrates, reacts to the on-or-off camera message.

In scenario # 1 and #2, the upgrade is usually given the day of the shoot.

In scenario #3, the upgrade will not be determined until the edited version is released. This means that even if you are photographed alone demonstrating the product but you are not featured in the final edit, you will not be upgraded.

In scenario #4, the upgrade can be determined on the set or during the edit session, with the final version determining if the upgrade is appropriate. There is such a thing as a "foreground background" meaning that you must meet all the requirements of scenario #4 to be upgraded.

If you are upgraded on a commercial, you may also be entitled to holdings fees when a spot is used beyond the initial thirteen week cycle. Also, additional compensation is due the performer if the commercial is aired on cable.

Singers and dancers can also be upgraded from background to principal. For dancers, the rule maintained is that if you are choreographed or directed by anyone, you are upgraded. If you are told to just "dance" or "make up your steps" you are considered background. With singers there are a number of factors that are judged on a case by case basis, with the entire performance being judged for the upgrade. Some of the conditions that are considered when determining an upgrade include:

☆ How the audition for the singers was described (did the production company ask for professional or trained singers?)

☆ How much rehearsal is necessary to perform.

If you are asked to harmonize or memorize special lyrics you may be upgraded while if the song you are asked to sing is a melody everyone would know, (like "Happy Birthday") your performance may be considered background work. All singers definitely should discuss each situation with their agent and the union which negotiated the contract.

If you have questions about your upgrade eligibility all concerns must be submitted within six months of working. If you are upgraded during an edit session, the statue of limitations begins on the first air date of the commercial.

If you feel you have performed principal work but were only paid as a background extra, contact your local Screen Actors Guild.

Downgrades and Outgrades

Just as you can be upgraded, you can also be downgraded or outgraded. As long as your face remains in the final edit of a commercial, you will receive residuals and remain a principal. However if you are downgraded or outgraded you will not. Here is the situation:

☆ Downgrades occur when your face is edited out of the commercial, but an image of you in some form remains. If you are downgraded from the commercial, you must be notified by the ad agency and be paid an additional session fee. No residuals are paid when timely notice is given. The definition of timely is within the thirteen week cycle.

☆ Outgrades occur when ALL of your performance has been eliminated from the commercial. This includes both your image, your voice and any soundtrack in which you had participated. Again, the ad agency must inform the performer in writing of the outgrade and when timely notice is delivered in writing, no residuals are due the performer.

Chapter 26

Fashion Modeling Information

"Be the Star You are!"

Supermodels can earn millions of dollars! Many teenage girls dream of becoming the next world hit, traveling to exotic locals to shoot magazine covers, commercials, and films. How do you get into this life?

Talent scouts are everywhere so you could just be lucky. Christy Turlington was riding horseback with her sister at age 16 when spotted by a photographer, Claudia Schiffer was dancing in Germany at a disco when an agent discovered her. However luck isn't the easiest route. A more conventional route is to send your photograph to a respected and top New York agency or go in person on their open call days. Nikki Taylor's mom sent photos to New York as soon as Nikki's braces came off at age 14.

What are agents looking for? Every year the look changes, but natural is definitely in at the moment. That means when you meet the agent, wear no make-up, no gussied up hair, no dangling accessories. Form fitting clothing makes it easier to assess the body, but that does not mean sexy. If you are asked to pose nude, refuse and run fast. That doesn't happen with legitimate agents or photographers.

The optimal age for fashion models is 17, some agencies like girls as young as 14 so that they can be trained their way. If you are over 22 you are probably over the hill. (There are exceptions to every rule, Lauren Hutton is well over 50 and still going strong) For women, the average height is 5'9" and above and for men 6' and above, however some agencies will take women 5'7" and above. (Kate Moss is only 5'7") Standard measurements are 34-24-34 with some variables. If you are overweight, this is not the place for you, try commercial print or acting which has no height and weight requirements. Long legs, very shapely without cellulite, high cheekbones, full lips, wide set eyes, and a long neck are fashionable. Agents are not looking for crossed eyes, thin hair, bad skin, wrinkled eyes, short legs, heavy bottoms, or big breasts with uneven bodily proportions.

Beginning pay is $150 per hour assuming you have pound the pavement and are getting booked for runway and print ads. Average pay for advertisements is about $3500 per day with catalog work being between $1250 and $2500. Obviously supermodels demand $15,000-$25,000 or more per day. One model, Kyle MacLachlan, was quoted as saying, "I don't get out of bed unless I'm earning $10,000 for the day." For fashion shows, models earn about $200 per hour or whatever the designer is willing to pay. Most agencies in San Francisco book their models for $200 for a formal show of one and half hours with each half hour at $125 per hour. Informal shows of 2 hours length are usually around $225.00. Lingerie and bathing suit rates are double with fittings, rehearsal, prep, travel time, make-up time and mini shows being additional fees. Rates vary by city and location, so always ask.

Difficult personalities, tantrum throwing, complicated personal lives, jealous boyfriends or girlfriends, drug or alcohol abuse, unprofessional behavior can all destroy a modeling career just the same as any career. Although you may be modeling part time, you must be fully committed to become successful. Even with complete commitment, success can be fleeting. The odds of getting chosen or being discovered are astronomical. The New York Agency, Elite, sees about 50,000 potential models every year. They will test about 100 and chose only about 30 for representation. Almost as difficult as the lottery to win! If you are petite (under 5'4") or a Plus model, there are fashion opportunities, but not in the big leagues. Most of the agencies listed have fashion divisions for children, petites, plus, and high fashion.

There are a few legitimate model searches each year. You may want to contact any of the following:

☆ International Modeling and Talent Association holds a convention in July in New York and in Los Angeles in January. Phone 602-997-4907

☆ Elite's Look of the Year contest takes place every September. Applications appear in Teen magazine. Phone 800-6-MATRIX

☆ Ford's Supermodel of America contest has regional June events then finals in August. Various magazines publish applications. Phone 212-308-7927

☆ Modeling Association of America International has a spring convention in New York. Phone 212-753-1555

Top Fashion Modeling Agencies

Listed below are addresses, phone numbers and open call times for top agencies in New York and San Francisco. Agents change, so please telephone in advance to assure that open call times/addresses are still current.

NEW YORK:	**Open Call times**
Elite Model Management 111 East 22nd Street New York, New York 10010 212-529-9700	Mon-Thurs 9:30am- 10:00am
Ford Agency 344 East 59th Street New York, New York 10022 212-753-6500	Wed. 3:00pm-4:00pm
Bethann Management Co. 36 N. Moore Street New York, New York 10013 212-925-2153	Send photos/SASE only
Next 115 East 57th Street New York, New York 10022 212-832-6403	Wed. 10:00am-11:00am

Click

1st Wed. noon-1:00pm

881 Seventh Avenue
New York, New York 10019
212-315-2200

Wilhelmina

Tues.-Thurs. 10-10:30am

300 Park Avenue South
New York, New York 10010
212-473-4610

Women

send photos/SASE
only

107 Greene Street, 2nd floor
New York, New York 10012
212-334-7480

Paris/USA

Thurs. 5:00pm-6:00pm

470 Park Avenue South
New York, New York 10010
212-683-9040

Metropolitan Model Management

Wed. 10:00am-11:00am

Union Square West
New York, New York 10003
212-989-0100

IT Models

Tues. 2:00-4:00pm

251 Fifth Avenue
New York, New York 10016
212-481-7220

IMG

Thurs. 10:30-11:00am

170 fifth Avenue
New York, New York 10010
212-627-0400

Company Management

Tues.-Thurs. 4:00-
4:30pm

270 Lafayette Street
New York, New York 10012
212-226-7000

SAN FRANCISCO

The San Francisco Agencies, with the exception of City Models, are franchised by SAG/AFTRA.

Boom Models and Talent   Tues./Thurs. 1-3pm
2324 3rd Street, #223
San Francisco, Ca. 94107
415-626-6591

City Models   Send photo/SASE only
123 Townsend Street, Suite 510
San Francisco, Ca. 94107
415-546-3160

Stars, the Agency   Tues. 2:00pm-4:00pm

23 Grant St 4th floor
San Francisco, Ca. 94108
415-421-6272

Look Agency   Mon. 2:00pm-4:00pm
166 Geary Blvd. #1406
San Francisco, Ca. 94108
415-781-2841

Marla Dell Talent   Send photo/SASE only
2124 Union Street
San Francisco, Ca. 94123
415-563-9213
(specializes in children's fashion)

Generations Model/Talent Agency   Send photo/SASE only
350 Townsend Street, Suite 408
San Francisco, Ca. 94107
415-349-0370
(specializes in children's fashion)

Average Model Rates Overveiw

One hour minimum on all photo shoots.

Photo shoots: Adults $150-200 per hour

Kids $75-$150 per hour

Pre-print fittings: 1/4 hourly rate

Travel time, outside of city: 1/2 hourly rate, round trip

Overtime: time + 1/2 for shoots before 9:00am and
 after 6:00pm

Fit Modeling: $75-$175 per hour

Back-up baby Rate: 1/2 shoot rate if not used

Sizes for Fit Modeling for Children

Children must fit exactly these sizes in order to be considered.

Size	Height
0-3 mon.	24″
3-6 mon.	24″-26.5″
6-9 mon.	26.5″-28″
12 mon.	28.5″-30.5″
18 mon.	31″-33″
18-24 mo.	33.5″-34.5″
2T	34.75-37″
3 T	37″-39.5″″
4T	39.5″-40.5″
4	40″-42.510
5	43″-46″
6	46.5″-47.5″
6X	48″-49″
7	49″-51″
8	52″-54.5″
10	55″-59″
12	59.5″-62″
14	62″-64″

The Fashion Show

There are basically three types of fashion shows: informal, formal and a combination of the two.

The Informal Fashion Show is usually held in a casual atmosphere such as a restaurant or store. It is loosely structured with any number of models mingling with guests and clientele discussing the merchandise. There is no commentary or staging or even a runway.

The Formal Fashion Show is structured and is usually on a runway or elevated stage. Often the show has been rehearsed and choreographed. It is augmented with commentary which details the originality and special aspects of the garment.

The Combination Show formally exhibits the clothing and accessories and informally discusses the finer points with the interested parties in attendance.

Fashion Show Runway Preparation

1. Arrive promptly at least half an hour before show time.
2. Be dressed and made up with full show make-up.
3. Have all your necessary accessories and props.
4. Always have a totebag with the essentials for a show with you.
5. Hang clothes in order of showing with name or marker on each hanger. Unbutton, unsnap, unhook, unzip the clothing. Tape the bottom of the shoes with masking tape. Check pants for correct hemline. If not, tape to the proper length for you.
6. Check for hanging tags. Tuck them in, pin them or use masking tape. Remove tags only as a last resort and tuck in a pocket.
7. Check each outfit for the total "show look". Make

sure you have everything together…shoes, earrings, bracelets, necklace, rings, etc.

8. Set up your accessories and props in order of show performance.

9. Don't use perfumes or after shave as the smell lingers in clothing. Watch for body odors. Use rubbing alcohol for perspiration and do use body shields and deodorants.

10. Make sure you have the information for each outfit in order. This is the outfit info sheet.

11. Keep brush, comb, pins, tape, scissor, tissues, towel, and make-up close by for quick touch ups.

12. Practice your walks and routines.

13. Before you get in front of the audience, know your clothing and create a personality and gait style.

14. After dressing do NOT sit, eat, smoke, or drink. Never bring food or beverages except water into the dressing area.

15. Always be ready in your complete outfit five minutes before show time.

16. Hang personal wardrobe in a separate location away from store merchandise.

17. Visualize a fun performance. Enjoy the show!

After the Show!

1. Check that all garments are hung correctly on the correct hangers and placed in the correct bags.

2. If there has been any damage to wardrobe report it immediately.

3. Put all tags properly in place on the right items

4. Return borrowed props and accessories.

5. Leave your area clean

6. Say "thank you" to everyone involved. Smile.

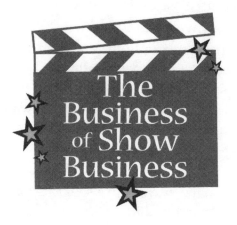

Chapter 27

Scams

"When one bases his life on principle, 99 percent of his decisions are already made. "
Unknown

Watch Out!

Starstyle Cue: If it sounds too good to be true, it usually is!

With that said, know that scams targeting the entertainment industry are on the rise. Children now comprise about 14% of Screen Actors Guild membership. With more children on television, ordinary people see stars in their eyes and big money by getting into acting and modeling. As a result, scams and scum operations abound for all ages. Everyone needs to be an informed consumer. People get drawn to these so called "agencies" by the hype: false promises of fame, fortune, entrance to talent agents, and non-existent movie parts. Some companies are not exactly scams, but they are definitely not part of the entertainment industry. Talent placement companies are proliferating, aggressively marketing to young wannabe actors and models stating that their purpose is to help performers secure a union franchised agent. Prices for this service including a package of photos (which are usually useless) and a few classes (of unknown quality) range in price from $800 to $10,000. Some of these "agencies" charge an additional lifetime commission on any work secured at any time with anyone of 5% or more. Some try to legitimize their business by contracting with well-known personalities. Unfortunately many of these operations are not illegal, only useless and a complete waste of time and money.

The ads for these companies are fairly standard stating: "Be a model or actor. New faces wanted, no experience necessary, will train, get great jobs in TV, movies, commercials, and magazines." Some companies go to county fairs, beauty pageants, school events and hand out cards or have drawings. (Of course, in the drawings everyone wins by getting a "free audition" where you end up being told what classes you must buy). Some companies run ads telling people to come try out for extra parts and charge a fee to be in the movie. These are called advance fee scams and they are the most frequent complaints heard in district attorney offices. They are based on false pretenses of promises without delivery of goods. It is a misdemeanor to guarantee a job and not give one.

People of all ages get drawn in by the hype. The first mistake is making the return phone call and the second is making the appointment "just to check it out!" Once in the door, these people are first class salespersons intent on making sure you sign the contract. The interview goes something like this: "My goodness, you are absolutely perfect for this business. If only you had been with us last week, we had the biggest commercial we could have cast you in, and you would have earned several thousand dollars. We sure don't want you to miss another opportunity. Now, you'll need a portfolio of photographs to get going and we recommend a few classes. Because we really want to represent you and make you money, we are going to give you a big discount on fees if you sign the contract today. Instead of $3500 for everything, you'll only pay $2500. Now sign right here and we'll make you a supermodel!"

Reading that paragraph makes me want to vomit and I know you are saying that scenario would never happen to you. Let me tell you something. Most of my clients found me only after already having spent at least $2500 for classes and portfolios they didn't need. And several of my longtime clients, after being solicited by these firms, were actually tempted to give these scams a try. The TV, radio, and newspaper advertisements are enticing. I was driving down the road the other day and on came a very upbeat, exciting radio commercial for a new "talent agency" that was seeking future stars for modeling and acting. It sounded so thrilling and I knew the ad would sucker in thousands of hopefuls. I called to get the information to warn my clients. Naturally, the person on the other end of the phone "could tell by my voice that I was a natural and would definitely become one of their top talent." It was recommended to me to come in immediately for my interview. As I probed a bit deeper, I was hesitantly informed that "yes, there may be a few classes I should take and of course I'd want to shoot photographs with their photographer who was a world renowned professional, but that they would definitely give me a discount because it was "obvious" I had star quality."" I hung up absolutely sick to my stomach knowing that so many people would buy into this hogwash.

What can you do to protect yourself? Arm yourself with information. Get a coach who works in this business that you totally trust. Ask people who are working as performers in the industry for a recommendation. Don't read the want ads or listen to commercials that advertise "Be a model or just look like one", etc. etc. Don't get involved with any agency that is not franchised by Screen Actors Guild or AFTRA. Franchised agencies are not allowed to advertise. If a company comes soliciting you, chances are it is a scam. In general, it is necessary for the talent to discover the agent, not the other way around. Never sign a contract on the spot. Use the excuse that your spouse, attorney, parent, whomever must review and approve before signing. If someone wants you today, they'll want you tomorrow.

If an agency asks for a fee up front, RUN. As has been written in many places in this book, legitimate talent agencies make their money from gross commissions only on work they have secured for you after the check is received from the client. No dollars or commissions or fees of any sort exchange hands before a job is completed.

Most of all, remember there are only two guarantees in life: death and taxes. Being promised or guaranteed work is a false claim and a definite sign of a scam. You don't need to spend money on lots of modeling classes to learn to walk, talk, and chew gum. Usually a one day runway workshop will give you all the information you'll need. Make-up application can be taught in a few hours. For acting, you want to make sure you are training under the tutelage of a working actor, not someone who has only taken acting classes. Acting is an on-going profession.

If you feel that you may be involved with a company that is not on the up and up, contact the Department of Consumer Affairs or your local district attorney's office. Scams have been around since the beginning of silent films. As long as there are people who have dreams of being the next Matt Damon, Gweneth Paltrow, Brad Pitt, or Britney Spears, there will be operations out there to promise you the moon. In order to become a star, you'll need to keep your feet and head on the ground!

<u>Beware! Be smart! Don't get bamboozled!</u>

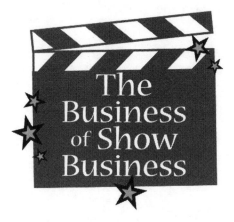

Chapter 28

Other Avenues to Hollywood

"Life is not based on the answers we receive, but on the questions we ask."

There are numerous other roads to stardom! Besides hundreds of jobs behind the camera lens, there is a myriad of other performing opportunities. You can be a voice over artist, a dancer, singer, musician, stunt person, combat expert, animal handler, or even just submit your home or business as a location for a shoot.

In this chapter I will address a few of the most lucrative professions.

Voice-overs

Doing voice-over work is a big business. Voice-overs are used in radio, television, film, CD Rom, and all phases of the entertainment industry. Voice-over is when your voice does the work and your body is not seen. This work has its advantages: it doesn't matter what you look like or how you dress for the audition, the only important factor is how well you can bring character to your voice. Although it sounds easier than on camera acting, it is actually more difficult to break into the voice-over business. The best advice is to take a private class or workshop from a professional voice-over coach. What you will need to market yourself will be a professionally produced and packaged voice tape and/or CD. What to put on the tape is best handled by the pros. You can practice your vocal skills by reading out loud, especially advertisements, and by taping yourself and listening to your presentation. Currently there is a tremendous need for bilingual or multilingual talent who have authentic accents and dialects.

There are voice over coaches all over the United States but my two favorite choices are listed below. These women are considered icons in our industry and have won numerous awards for their work. Besides being sought after voice over talent in their own right, they know how to teach others to achieve the dream.

Lucille Bliss: 415-824-8186
Susan McCollom: 415-956-3878

Stage Combat

Choreographed fights, including fighting with weapons, are the basis of stage combat. The Society of American Fight Directors (SAFD) recognizes 31 fight directors nationally with San Francisco boasting four of them. SAFD also has 54 certified teachers and about 2500 recognized actor combatants. Knowledge of combat skills is essential for the safety of actors who are required to work with swords, rapiers, scimitars, quarter staffs and plain old punches! A credentialed fight director and rehearsal time on the set ensures that a fight is safer and more believable. Actors who are trained to handle weapons have the edge when it comes to casting. The skills learned in a stage combat workshop will increase awareness and give experience in handling weapons that will serve an actor for years.

Certified Teachers:
Academy of the Sword
(Richard Lane, Bob Borwick, Kit Wilder)
587 Lisbon St.
San Francisco, Ca. 94112
415-957-3622

American Academy of Stage Combat
(Larry Henderson)
259 Elysian Fields Drive
Oakland, Ca. 94605
510-632-0938

Dueling Arts International
(Gregory Hoffman)
PO Box 17257
Stanford, Ca. 94309
650-564-6040

Dexter Fidler
635 Judah St.
San Francisco, Ca. 94122
415-564-6040

Stunts

They jump out of airplanes, fall down flights of stairs, drive stagecoaches over canyons, hurl out of ten story buildings on fire, and execute car chases that could spell disaster. Yet, they are not daredevils. These are the cautionary, rare breed of men and women of stunt work. They are a group of highly skilled professionals who prepare and choreograph each stunt with precision clarity with an eye towards safety. They work as a team, are extremely well trained and highly skilled athletes that don't leave anything to chance.

Because of their expertise and experience, movie-goers enjoy thrills on screen that are rarely witnessed in real life.

In my early years of acting, I performed numerous small stunts. As an athlete, I was agile, quick, and precise. My resume included sky diving, scuba diving, white water rafting, horseback riding, most field sports, and the ability to drive all types of vehicles, including trucks, tractors, and motorcycles. I was often called upon for stunt scenes and I was jubilant to be cast. I drove fast cars and skidded across freeways, did loop de loops in biplanes, was knocked down an escalator by a leading star, and rode motorcycles on the edge of precipices. I was injured a few times, but I loved the thrill. Little did I know that stunt work is a specialty, a skill that smart people train for with diligence and prudence. Thank goodness I woke up one day and understood that stunts need to be performed by professionally trained stunt people. Looking back I acknowledge my stupidity in taking the risks I took. I survived, thankfully, but many untrained people who try stunts have not.

If you are athletic or already are an expert equestrian, pilot, motorcycle racer, martial artist, mountain climber or whatever and are interested in pursuing a career in stunts,

I suggest you contact one of the stunt associations or stunt schools listed below. The life you save may be your own.

☆ Stunt Players Directory:
　http://www.stuntplayers.com

☆ Stuntmen's Association:
　http://www.stuntmen.com

☆ Professional Drivers Association:
　http://www.stuntplayers.com/pro-drivers

☆ United Stuntman's Association:
　http://www.stuntschool.com/school.htm

☆ Frogmen Unlimited:
　http://www.frogmen.com

☆ Stunts Unlimited :
　http://stuntsunlimited.com

☆ United Stuntwomen's Association:
　http://www.usastunt.com

Make Your Home a Star!

Would you like to get your home in a movie, commercial, or print ad? Homes and gardens are always in demand from run down slum houses to high society penthouses. Cutting edge designs, unique wall treatments and views are all valued in the entertainment industry as possible locations. Victorians, warehouses, barns, Arts and Craft cottages to chalets are always wanted.

What does it pay? Standard rates are anywhere from $500 to $5000 per day depending on the location, job, and length of the shoot. Print jobs may take a few hours whereas a commercial may be a few days and movies may be three to four months.

What do you need to do? Take at least 36 color photos of both interior and exterior of your location including wide angles and close-ups. For exterior shots, walk across the street and shoot from a distance. Make sure to take close-ups of special details such as gates, waterfalls, aviaries, ponds, pools, or large lawns. For interiors, shoot every room of the house from different angles and at different times of the day. Include shots of all architectural details such as moldings, doors, fireplaces, wine cellars, high windows, staircases, marble, wood floors, etc. Write a complete description of your property with dimensions and send if off to local film commissions to put on file for location scouts to peruse. Make sure to include your name, address, and phone numbers.

Are there pitfalls to allowing your home or gardens to be used for shoots? You bet there are. The money can be great but you must be prepared for complete upheaval of your lifestyle and a fair amount of property damage. Make sure that you have increased your homeowner's insurance and that you get a contract from the production company which will also provide insurance coverage. Many strangers will be coming to your space in addition to miles and miles of cables, lights, dollies, ramps, cameras, trucks, vans, generators, honey wagons, trailers, and portable potties. Although most film companies put things back the way they found them and repair any damages, you will definitely have some wear and tear including scratches and fingerprints. Therefore you must be doing it for more than the money. There are occasions when your home actually gets improvements like a swimming pool, pond, or tennis court and sometimes you'll get hired to work as an extra for an additional $50 per day.

If interested, send your information to your local city or state film commission. Listed are a few California Film Commission offices.

Berkeley Film Office
1834 University Ave.
Berkeley, Ca. 94703

San Francisco Film
Commission
401 Van Ness Ave. #417
San Francisco, Ca. 94102

Oakland Film Commission
1333 Broadway
Oakland, Ca. 94612

Sonoma County Film
Commission
5000 Roberts Lake Road
Rohnert Park, Ca. 94928

San Jose Film Commission
333 West San Carlos St. #1000
San Jose, Ca. 95110

California Film
Commission
6922 Hollywood Blvd.
Hollywood, Ca. 90028

Animals on Parade

All my life I have raised animals and have a special way of working with them. Having grown up on a farm, I was used to not only the normal household pets like dogs and cats, but horses, cows, sheep, goats, pigs, rabbits, geese, ducks, deer, and chickens...just to name a few. In fact, I raised chickens and sold the eggs as a 4-H'er for nine years to earn enough money to fund my college education. For several years I was California's Grand Champion rooster raiser! Ironically this title helped land me several prime acting jobs as an adult.

When I began acting I wasn't about to give up my critters. I wanted my animal pals to play with me. So I shot photos of the various animals and gave them to my agent "just in case they ever got a call for….(fill in the type of animal)". The agents got the calls and the producers began to recognize that they could count on a Cynthia Brian animal for their shoot. Over the years my dogs, rabbits, ducks, goats, geese, pig, chickens, and exotic birds have all worked with me in various print and TV jobs. And we BOTH got paid. For print, the going rate for my animals was one half my hourly fee and for television it was whatever was negotiated. We always had a wonderful time and we made money that could pay for the upkeep. My pets were not trained to do tricks, they were just always very loving, docile, easy to work with family pets.

Today, there are agencies that book only animals. Most animal agencies are always looking for well-trained, well disciplined animals for work in commercials, print, and live performances. Most agencies want to see a video tape, pictures, and resume of the skills of the animal. Some agents have training centers as well. While most of the big jobs will go to professional animal handlers, it is worth a try if you have a special animal to register with a professional agency. For animal agencies in your area, consult your local production guide, or do a search on the internet. Make sure to ask around and get referrals or references. If you already have a talent agent you might try doing what I did and give them photos of your animals with you. At the minimum, inform your agent of your ability with animals.

My husband has also been a collector of vintage cars and for awhile the joke in our family was that a member of our household was always modeling or acting…sometimes it was me or the children, many times the animals, and once in awhile our cars. But that is a story for another book!

Animal Agencies

This is not a comprehensive list of agencies that represent animals, nor is this list an endorsement of the agencies mentioned. Please refer to your local film directory for legitimate agencies in your area. Always get references.

All Star Animals:
707-585-7667 or 800-787-3647

Animal Actors International:
http://www.animal-actors.com

Animal Connection:
http://www.animal-connection.com

Amazing Animals Actor:
http://www.amazinganimalactors.com

Bow Wow Productions:
800-926-9969

Hollywood Animals:
http://www.hollywoodanimals.com

T.I.G.E.R.S:
http://www.tigers-animal-actors.com
(exotic animals)

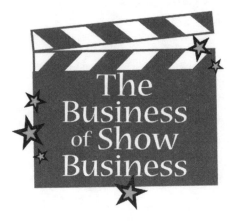

Chapter 29

Talking Taxes

*"I'd rather learn from one bird how to sing than
teach ten thousand stars how not to dance."*
                                        ee cummings

In the entertainment industry, taxpayers are
involved in three primary activities:
- ☆ performing
- ☆ searching for work
- ☆ enhancing job skills

All deductible expenses must have a direct and specific
correlation to the work performed, the auditioning and
interviewing process or the training and education of the

entertainer. Expenses can not be deducted for ordinary and general purposes.

I am not an accountant nor am I a tax expert, so I offer this chapter as information only with the disclaimer that I advise you to seek advice from your personal financial advisor. Get a good accountant and talk to him/her about what is allowed for you. Don't ask another actor or friend. You need a specialist with all the new laws being implemented each year. Each person's situation is different so the answer a specialist gives to your best friend may not be the same advice for you. In other words, GET YOUR OWN ACCOUNTANT.

These are my tips, based on experience.

Prepare your taxes early. Keep accurate and clear records of your daily activities. Keep all receipts which pertain to the business of show business.

By filing early, if Uncle Sam owes you money you'll get it sooner. If you owe taxes you have until April 15 to find the money you owe. The money can remain in the bank earning interest until tax time. Get started early on taxes. A penny saved is a penny earned. Make sure to invest in a ROTH IRA account for your retirement. Currently you can deposit $3000 –3500 depending on your age and that amount most likely will increase in the coming years. A SEP allows more. When you retire you will be glad you have some savings!

Here is a list of the most common general business deductions for acting and modeling. Please check with your tax specialist for your particular tax needs:

☆ advertising and publicity

☆ accompanist and audition expenses

☆ agent's commissions and manager's fees

☆ answering service and answering machine

- ☆ coaching and lessons for performance
- ☆ entertainment for business purposes (records must indicate who, where, when, and why)
- ☆ gifts for business (limit of $25 per person per year)
- ☆ parking and transportation and bridges
- ☆ acting, dance and performing art classes
- ☆ office supplies, stationery, postage
- ☆ make-up and cosmetics
- ☆ photography
- ☆ printing of photos and resumes
- ☆ professional equipment (tape recorder, VCR, typewriter, computer, printer, answering machine, FAX)
- ☆ studio and equipment rentals
- ☆ tax preparation costs
- ☆ legal fees
- ☆ portfolio costs
- ☆ telephone, pager (business calls only)
- ☆ travel including lodging, airfare, transportation, meals
- ☆ trade publications, books, scripts, and sheet music
- ☆ Union dues and initiation fees
- ☆ costume, laundry, and cleaning (wardrobe for some jobs)
- ☆ body care, including haircuts, facials, manicures, etc. (certain situations)
- ☆ role research: theatre and concert tickets, movies, videos, cable TV
- ☆ donations
- ☆ auto (mileage, oil, repairs, insurance)

General Reminders

✮ Your unemployment benefits are now fully taxable.

✮ Income averaging is no longer allowed.

✮ Medical expenses must exceed 7.5% of adjusted gross income to be deductible.

✮ Only 50% of the cost of business meals and entertainment is deductible.

✮ Business use of the home requires very careful documentation. The space must be exclusively used for business purposes and income must be generated.

✮ There are now only two tax brackets for most people.

✮ Wardrobe expenses are not deductible if the clothes can be worn for general personal wear.

✮ Mileage reimbursement is 36.5 cents per mile.

✮ Keeping in shape is not deductible unless physical attributes are so intertwined with the performing roles.

HAIR STYLING/MAKE-UP: Although our appearance is one of our greatest assets, the IRS now considers anything regarding looks to be personal. This means the deductions have been narrowed. Any hair cuts, styles, colors, make-up, facials, manicures, etc. for general purposes are considered personal and therefore not deductible. If you need to purchase special make-up for a shoot or have your hair or nails done for a particular job, this item will be deductible as long as the production company does not reimburse you for the costs.

GYMS, BODY CONDITIONING: The same principles apply here as with hair and make-up. In the past personal trainers, gyms, workouts, exercise equipment were all deductible. Now the only deduction for such activities is if they are for a specific job or you make your living by your bodily attributes, for example, you are a bathing suit or lingerie model or a muscle man like Arnold or Sylvester.

MOVIES, VIDEOS, THEATRE: In the old days we were allowed to write all our ticket costs off as an education expense. Now the IRS looks at these things as pure entertainment with no educational value for the business. Again, the only way these items will be deductible is if you are studying the performance of an actor, or directing techniques of a director for a specific upcoming job or audition. In this scenario, the IRS will allow only a percentage of the actual ticket cost.

IRCSS179: You may deduct 100% of the cost of any business equipment (except an auto) purchased for business use. Certain restrictions are applied to autos and equipment purchases may not exceed an allowance of $17,500 with documentation.

The IRS is tightening up its grip on our industry. As always, it is best to keep accurate records, ask for receipts, keep canceled checks, and to consult with a tax accountant regarding your particular situation as all taxpayers have different circumstances.

Tax law is gray, never black and white so inter-pretations differ. Remember the three buzz words of the IRS: "ordinary and necessary." If an expense item represents a typical payment during the normal course of business, then that expense item by law, is deductible. If you spend a dollar to earn a dollar, it is deductible. It is that simple!

VOLUNTEER INCOME TAX ASSISTANCE: Free tax preparation assistance is available through SAG, AFTRA, and EQUITY in New York, Hollywood, and Chicago. Volunteers are ready to help you file. Call:

Chicago	(312)641-0405
New York	(212)921-2548
Hollywood	(323)856-6605

Remember: Be prepared. Be honest. Get a specialist to help you. Keep records. Save receipts. Document everything!

Chapter 30

Suggested Reading List

"Help each other to be happy.
Never mind if help be small.
Giving a little is far better
Than giving none at all."
Father Patrick McGrath

Bookstores

These bookstores can order any acting/modeling books for you.

Samuel French
7623 Sunset Blvd
Hollywood, Ca. 90046
213) 876-0570

Drama Books Shops
723 7th Avenue
New York, 10019
(212) 944-0595

Samuel French Bookstore
11963 Ventura Boulevard
Studio City, CA 91604
818) 762-0535

Larry Edmunds Bookstore
6644 Hollywood Boulevard
Hollywood, CA 90028
(213) 463-3273

Stage and Screen Book Club
www.joinstagenscreen.com

Hollywood Creative
Directory (for film directories)
1024 N. Orange Drive
Hollywood, Ca. 90038
http://hcdonline.com
800-815-0503

Books

About Your Career

1. Your Film Acting Career by MK Lewis and Rosemary Lewis (Crown Publishing)
2. Acting in Television Commercials for Fun and Profit by Squire Fridell (Harmony Books)
3. How to get work and make money in commercials and modeling by Cecily Hunt (Van Nostrand Reinhold Co.)
4. How to get into Commercials by Vangie Hayes (Barnes and Noble Books)
5. True and False: Heresay and Common Sense for the Actor by David Mamet (Vintage)

Auditioning

1. How to Audition by Gordon Hunt (Harper and Row)
2. Audition by Michael Shurtleff (Walker and Co.)

Acting

Books by Constantin Stanislavski (Theatre Arts Books)
1. An Actor's Handbook
2. An Actor Prepares
3. Creating a Role
4. Building a Character

Other Authors:

5. Respect for Acting by Uta Hagen (Macmillan Publishing
6. To the Actor by Michael Checkhov (Harper and Row)
7. The Stanislavski System by Sonia Moore (Viking)
8. No Acting, Please by Eric Morris and Joan Hotchkis
    (Spelling Publications)
9. The Audition Book by Ed Hooks (Backstage Books)
10. Sanford Meisner on Acting by Sanford Meisner (Vintage)

General

1. Actors on Acting by Toby Cole and Helen Chinoy (Crown
    Publishers)
2. Improvisation for the Theatre by Viola Spolin (University of
    Chicago Press)
3. Gaffers, Grips, and Best Boys by Eric Taub
4. The AFTRA-SAG Young Performers Handbook (available to
    members at SAG/AFTRA offices)
5. Swashbuckling: the art of stage combat and theatrical
    Swordplay by Richard Lane (Proscenium Press)
6. A Blow by Blow Guide to Sword Fighting in the Renaissance
    Style by Gregory Hoffman
7. Be the Star You Are! 99 Gifts for Living, Loving, Laughing,
    and Learning to Make a Difference by Cynthia Brian
    (Ten Speed Press)
8. Meditations for Actors by Carra Robertson (Dablon Books)
9. The Reel Directory (Lynetta Freeman call 707-933-9935)
10. What Color is Your Parachute? By Richard Nelson Bolles
    (Ten Speed)

Voice

1. Freeing the Natural Voice by Kristin Linklater (Drama Books
2. The Use and Training of the Human Voice by Arthur Lessac
    (Drama Books)

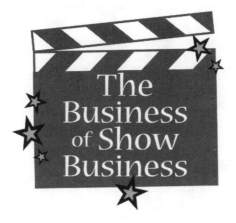

Chapter 31

Other Entertainment Industry Unions, Organizations, And Studios

"They are ill discoverers that think there is no land, when they see nothing but sea."
Francis Bacon

Entertainment Unions

ACTRA - Alliance of Canadian Television and Radio Artists - A National Organization of Canadian Performers Working in Film, Television, Video and all other Recorded Media.

AEA - Actors Equity Association - is the labor union representing actors and stage managers in the legitimate theatre in the United States. Equity negotiates minimum wages and working conditions, administers contracts, and enforces the provisions of its various agreements with theatrical employers.

AFM - American Federation of Musicians - The largest union in the world representing the professional interests of musicians.

AGMA - American Guild of Musical Artists - The labor organization that represents the men and women who create America's operatic, choral and dance heritage.

AGVA - American Guild of Variety Artists - present jurisdiction includes performers in Broadway, Off-Broadway, Cabaret productions, night club entertainers and theme park performers.

DGA - Director's Guild of America - Represents members in theatrical, industrial, educational and documentary films, as well as television live, filmed and taped radio, videos and commercials.

IATSE - International Alliance of Theatrical Stage Employees - Represents technicians, artisans and crafts persons in the entertainment industry, including live theater, film and television production.

Local 47-AFM - The Professional Musicians Local 47 is a 100-plus-year old labor organization representing over 9,000 local members. They act together to protect their mutual interests, to promote and conserve their craft, to agree on fair prices and conditions, and to enforce fair dealings in the profession. They combine their strength to do whatever we can do better collectively than we can do individually.

NABET-CWA Local 57 - National Association of Broadcast Employees & Technicians - Communications Workers of America

WGA - Writers Guild of America, East - Negotiates Minimum Basic Agreements with major producers of motion pictures and television programs as well as contracts for staff members at radio and television stations.

WGA - Writers Guild of America, West - Is the sole collective bargaining representative for writers in the motion picture, broadcast, cable, interactive and new media industries.

Industry Organization

AAAA - American Association of Advertising Agencies - AAAA is the national trade organization representing the advertising agency business. It is a management-oriented organization, offering its members the broadest feasible depth of information regarding the operation of advertising agencies, encompassing management, media, print and broadcast production, secondary research on advertising and marketing, international advertising and much more.

AAJA - Asian American Journalists Association - A non-profit organization with approximately 1,700 members in seventeen chapters nationwide and in Asia.

AFI - American Film Institute - The only national arts organization devoted to film, television and video, The American Film Institute serves as a point of national focus and coordination for the many individuals and institutions concerned with the moving image as art.

AIAS - Academy of Interactive Arts & Sciences - This not-for-profit organization will serve as a forum to: Promote and advance common interests in the worldwide interactive community, Recognize outstanding achievement in interactive content and the interactive community, Conduct an annual awards show and enhance the image and awareness of the interactive arts and sciences.

AICP - Association of Independent Commercial Producers - Members comprise companies that specialize in producing commercials, regardless of length, on various media — film, video, computer — for advertisers and agencies.

AMPAS - Academy of Motion Picture Arts & Sciences - Several kinds of information are available about the Academy, the Academy Awards, and the other programs and activities of the Academy and its affiliated organization, the Academy Foundation.

ASCAP - American Society of Composers, Authors and Publishers - Allows creators and publishers to receive payment for the use of their musical property and provides users of that music with easy and inexpensive legal access to the world's largest and most varied catalog of copyrighted music.

ATA - The Association of Talent Agents - is a nonprofit trade association composed of approximately 100 agency companies engaged in the talent agency business. The membership includes agencies of all sizes representing clients in the motion picture industry, stage, television, radio (including commercials) and literary work.

AWRT - American Women in Radio and Television - A national, non-profit organization dedicated to advancing women in the electronic media and related fields. Established in 1951, AWRT has local chapters throughout the United States that promote AWRT's mission: to advance the impact of women in the electronic media and allied fields, by educating, advocating and acting as a resource to members and the industry.

BMI - Source for the song titles, writers and publishers of the world's most popular music — the BMI repertoire — in a searchable database of millions of items, updated weekly, together with the Web's most complete fund of information for and about songwriting and music licensing.

EIC- Entertainment Industries Council, Inc. - To lead the entertainment industry in bringing it's power and influence to bear on health and social issues.

EIF - Entertainment Industry Foundation - The Entertainment Industry Foundation is still the heart and soul of the industry. It has maintained its historical commitment to coordinate the philanthropy of the entertainment industry to achieve maximum social impact in the community thanks to the generosity of the people who work in the industry.

HRTS - Hollywood Radio and Television Society - An organization of West Coast executives from the networks, stations, studios, producers, advertisers, ad agencies, cable companies, media companies, legal firms, publicity agencies, talent and management agencies, performers, services, suppliers and allied fields.

MCA-I - Media Communications Association-International - Serves the needsof accomplished visual communicators who work in corporate, organizational, and independent settings. It has 8000 members in over 100 chapters throughout the U.S.

Museum of Television and Radio - A unique institution with locations in both New York City and Los Angeles, its goal is to collect and make available to the public the finest collection of programs, and promote a greater appreciation of their artistic value, social impact, and historic importance.

NAB - National Association of Broadcasters - Represents the radio and television industries in Washington — before Congress, the FCC and federal agencies, the courts, and on the expanding international front. NAB provides leadership and its vast resources to our supporting members, to broadcasters at-large, and through ongoing public service campaigns to the American people.

NABJ - National Association of Black Journalists: mission is to strengthen ties among African-American journalists, promote diversity in newsrooms, honor excellence and outstanding achievement in the media industry, expand job opportunities and recruiting activities for established African-American journalists and students interested in the journalism field, and expand and balance the media's coverage of the African-American community and experience.

NAHJ - The National Association of Hispanic Journalists: is dedicated to the recognition and professional advancement of Hispanics in the news industry.

NARAS - National Academy of Recording Arts & Sciences - Dedicated to improving the quality of life and cultural condition for music and its makers. An organization of more than 11,000 musicians, producers and other recording professionals, The Recording Academy is internationally known for the GRAMMY® Awards.

NATAS – National Academy of Television Arts & Sciences - A non-profit corporation devoted both to the advancement of telecommunications arts and sciences and to fostering creative leadership in the telecommunications industry. Is also responsible for the annual Emmy Awards.

NATPE - National Association of Television Program Executives - Is the world's leading non-profit television programming and software association dedicated to the continued growth and success of the global television marketplace.

NCAC - National Coalition Against Censorship - an alliance of over 40 national non-profit organizations, including literary, artistic, religious, educational, professional, labor, and civil liberties groups. United by a conviction that freedom of thought, inquiry, and expression must be defended, we work to educate our own members and the public at large about the dangers of censorship and how to oppose it. NCAC strives to create a climate of opinion hospitable to First Amendment freedoms in the broader community.

NLGJA - National Lesbian and Gay Journalists Association - works from within the news industry to foster fair and accurate coverage of lesbian and gay issues and opposes newsroom bias against lesbians and gays and all other minorities.

RIAA - Recording Industry Association of America - The trade group promoting the vitality of U.S. recording companies.

RTNDA - Radio-Television News Directors Association: represents local and network news executives in broadcasting, cable and other electronic media in more than

30 countries. Through RTNDA's programs, publications, products and services, the association's members stay on top of trends in the electronic news industry, keep informed about technological innovations, expand their professional networks, stay in touch with issues affecting the industry and enhance their journalistic and news management skills.

Service Organizations

The Actors Fund of America - The Actors' Fund is for people on the stage and behind the scenes, in front of the camera and behind the lens. It's for agents and announcers, carpenters and clowns, actors and dancers, magicians and musicians, producers and free agents, stage hands and singers. People in film and theatre, TV, and radio, music, dance and opera, and the full spectrum of other entertainment media have always turned to The Actors' Fund when some personal or family crisis threatens their well-being.

AFTRA Health & Retirement Funds - Provides AFTRA members with the most current information regarding health and retirement benefits.

AFTRA-SAG Federal Credit Union – a credit union for AFTRA members

Career Transition for Dancers - The mission of Career Transition for Dancers is to empower current and former professional dancers with the knowledge and skills necessary to clearly define their career possibilities after dance, and to provide resources necessary to help make these possibilities a reality.

The Motion Picture & Television Fund - A major service organization promoting the well being of California's entertainment community. Health care and child care, retirement and social/charitable services are provided with compassion and respect for the dignity of the whole person. Particular emphasis is placed on the Motion Picture & Television Hospital, five health centers, financial assistance and community outreach programs, a retirement community and the Samuel Goldwyn Foundation Children's Center.

SAG Pension & Health Funds – Provides SAG members with the most current information regarding health and pension benefits

Singers and Musicians Organization

ACF: American Composers Forum - One of the largest composer-service organizations in the United States.

AFM: American Federation of Musicians - Union that represents professional musicians.

AFIM: Association for Independent Music - Organization that helps the independent music community through shared information & education.

AMC: The American Music Center - National service organization devoted exclusively to the greater field of contemporary American music.

AMG: All Music Guide - Database of recorded music.

ASCAP: American Society of Composers, Authors and Publishers – Performing rights society that licenses the public performance of members' copyrighted musical compositions and collects and distributes the license fees.

Billboard - The music industry's premiere news resource, covering all aspects of the music industry. Definitive source for sales figures, concert grosses and many other industry indices. Weekly listings of various Billboard charts; audio samples of chart hits; weekly previews of major music releases; a weekly trivia game; bonus chart facts and more.

BMI: Broadcast Music, Inc. - Performing rights organization that licenses the public performance of affiliates' copyrighted musical compositions and collects and distributes the license fees.

CMA: Country Music Association - Trade organization for Country Music.

CSUSA: Copyright Society of the USA - Organization that focuses on the gathering, dissemination and interchange of information concerning intellectual property rights.

Future of Music Coalition - Organization that addresses pressing music-technology issues and serves as a voice for musicians in Washington, D.C., where critical decisions are being made regarding musicians' intellectual property rights without a word from the artists themselves.

GMA: Gospel Music Association - Organization that supports, encourages and promotes the development of all forms of gospel music.

HFA: Harry Fox Agency - Organization that provides an information source, clearing house and monitoring service for licensing musical copyrights.

International Lyrics Server - Database searchable by song lyrics.

La Costa Music - Contains all kinds of how-to information, music industry trivia and forms.

MAP: Musicians Assistance Program - Organization that helps members of the music industry to receive treatment for drug and alcohol addiction, regardless of their financial condition.

MENC: The National Association for Music Education (formerly Music Educators National Conference) - Organization to advance music education.

MPA: Music Publishers' Association - Non-profit association addressing issues pertaining to music publishing with an emphasis on the issues relevant to the publishers of print music for concert and educational purposes.

MusiCares - Foundation was established in 1989 by the National Academy of Recording Arts and Sciences with the objective of focusing the attention and resources of the music industry on the health, human service and welfare needs of all music people. Provides assistance to music people in need of financial or other assistance.

NARAS: National Academy of Recording Arts & Sciences - Also known as the Recording Academy. Dedicated to improving the quality of life and cultural conditions for music and its makers. Produces the GRAMMY Awards.

NMC: National Music Foundation - Organization dedicated to American music and the people who create it through educational programs and performances and by providing retirement-related assistance to musicians and professionals from related fields.

NMPA: The National Music Publishers Association - Organization of American music publishers dedicated to the protection of music copyright across all media and national boundaries.

NSAI: The Nashville Songwriters Association International - Songwriters trade organization.

Official Copyright - Company that provides automated filing and protection products and services for intellectual property works and offers a direct gateway for online filing of copyrights.

RAC: Recording Artists Coalition - Advocacy group for recording artists.

RIAA: Recording Industry Association of America - Trade group that represents the U.S. recording industry.

SESAC - Performing rights organization that licenses the public performance of affiliates' copyrighted musical compositions and collects and distributes the license fees.

SGA: The Songwriters Guild of America - Songwriters organization.

Society of Singers - Nonprofit charity that helps professional vocalists worldwide in times of crisis. SOS provides emergency financial aid, case management, counseling and referral services. SOS is not a union, talent agency or employment service.

Sound Exchange - Organization comprised of large, medium and small recording companies, that licenses the public performance of sound recordings on digital channels like cable, satellite and the Internet and collects and distributes the license fees.

StarPolish - Free website that offers music industry advice, resources and information on current issues, as well as multi-tiered rewards and a grant program.

U.S. Copyright Office - Obtain updates on U.S. and international copyright laws. Forms and "how to" information can be found here.

Broadcast Network

ABC News
CBS News
NBC News
ABC - American Broadcasting Company
CBS - Columbia Broadcasting System
NBC - National Broadcasting Company
NPR - National Public Radio
PBS - Public Broadcasting System
FOX - The Fox Network
UPN - United Paramount Network
WB - Warner Brothers Network

Major Studio

Castle Rock Ent.
Comedy Central
Dreamworks SKG
Fox Broadcasting
HBO
MTV
Metro Goldwyn Mayer
Miramax
New Line Cinema
Nickelodeon

Paramount Studios
Showtime Network
Sony Pictures Ent.
Turner Entertainment
Twentieth Century Fox
Universal Studios
Viacom Ent
Walt Disney Co.
Warner Bros. Studios

Labor Organizations

AFL-CIO - Stated mission is to improve the lives of working families and to bring economic justice to the workplace and social justice to the nation.

DOL - Department of Labor - is charged with preparing the American workforce for new and better jobs, and ensuring the adequacy of America's workplaces. It is responsible for the administration and enforcement of over 180 federal statutes. These legislative mandates and the regulations produced to implement them cover a wide variety of workplace activities for nearly 10 million employers and well over 100 million workers, including protecting workers' wages, health and safety, employment and pension rights; promoting equal employment opportunity; administering job training, unemployment insurance and workers' compensation programs; strengthening free collective bargaining and collecting, analyzing and publishing labor and economic statistics.

LaborNet - supports human rights and economic justice for workers by providing labor news and information, comprehensive Internet services, training and web site design for union and labor organizations.

NLRB - National Labor Relations Board - is an independent Federal agency created in 1935 by Congress to administer the National Labor Relations Act, the basic law governing relations between labor unions and the employers whose operations affect interstate commerce.

Chapter 32

Web Sites

"Choose always the way that seems the best,
however rough it may be; custom will soon
render it easy and agreeable."
Pythagoras

Not everyone is web savvy yet, and many people still fear getting on line. I want to encourage you to get familiar with the benefits as many wonderful resources and vital information for a career in acting and modeling are available via the internet. Sites change rapidly so always seek the updated versions. I've listed a few of my favorite sites, but of course, I urge you to always use your own best judgement when taking the recommendations from a web site. Please let me know of your favorite sites and they'll be considered for future editions of this book.

Two sites for good career info operated by LA actors
http://www.actorsite.com
http://www.caryn.com/

Movie scripts
http://www.script-o-rama.com/table.shtml
http://www.alask.net

Extras:
http://www.extracast.com

Cooperative script service
http://www.newplays.com/liks.html

Crew listings:
http://www.crew-list.net

Tony Awards
http://www.tonys.org

TheatreBay Area/Callboard
http://www.theatrebayeara.org

Directors Guild of America
http://www.dga.org

Entertainment News Daily
http://www.entertainmentnewsdaily.com

Internet Movie Database
http://www.IMDB.com

SAG, natioanl offices
http://www.sag.org

AFTRA national offices
http://www.aftra.com

AFTRA/SAG office in SF
http://www.aftrasf.org

Backstage trade paper
http://www.backstage.com

Writers guild of Ameria
http://www.wga.org

Collection of theatre links
http://www.playbill.com

Bay area publication for casting
http://www.CastingConnection.com

Academy of Motion Picture Arts/Sciences
http://www.ampas.org

Show business articles/news
http://www.showbizdigest.com

Variety Trade publication
http://www.variety.com/

Beau Bonneau Casting, San Francisco
http://www.sfcasting.com

The Players Directory
http://www.playersdirectory.com

Shoptalk - News about the broadcasting business
http://www.shoptalk.com

Showbizwire
http://www.showbizwire.com/

Billboard:
http://www.billboard.com

The Players Directory:
http://www.playersdirectory.com

Daily Variety:
http://dailynews.yahoo.com/
headlines/entertainment/variety/
index.html

E!:
http://dailynews.yahoo.com/h/
en/eo/

Entertainment Weekly:
http://www.ew.com/ew/

Hollywood Reporter:
http://dailynews.yahoo.com/h/
en/bpihw/

LA Daily News:
http://
www.dailynewslosangeles.com/

LA Times:
http://www.latimes.com/
Muchmusic:
http://www.muchmusic.com

Motion Picture and TV Links:
http://www.mptv.com

**Motion Picture, TV, and Theatre
Directory for products and
services**:
http://www.mpe.net

New York Film and Video Guide:
http://www.nyfilmguide.com/

People:
http://people.aol.com

PR Newswire:
http://www.prnewswire.com

R & R:
http://www.rronline.com/

TV Shoptalk:
http://www.tvspy.com/
shoptalk.cfm

Rolling Stone:
http://www.rollingstone.com/

Showbiz Network - Source for cast-
and-crew requirements!
http://www.showbiznetwork.com

Stuntmen's Association
http://www.stuntmen.com

Starstyle® Productions
http://www.star-style.com

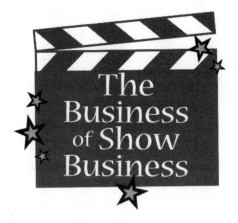

Chapter 33

It's Up to You!

"You can lead a horse to water, but you can't make him drink."

Author unknown

We have come to the end of The Business of Show Business. I hope you will find the information included herein pertinent to creating a career in a vocation of passion. Remember that no one can make you a star. Only you possess the power to create your own destiny. It has been my goal to guide you through the numerous doors of the entertainment industry. It is now up to you to walk right in and get the job. It may be frightening at first but the only way to know your limits is to over reach them. The great thing is not to play it safe.

In the middle of difficulty lies opportunity. Meet each challenge with courage and a sense of "I CAN do this." There are no failures in life as long as you are learning lessons. Success is just failure turned inside out. As I always tell my students and clients, "Failure is fertilizer!" Deem to do your best, and know that you won't win every time out, but each time you get a "no" you are just closer to a "yes". Keep going, and don't quit. Soon you'll be considered a professional. After all, an expert at anything was once a beginner.

So what are you waiting for? Get off the couch and go into action to make your dreams come true. You have a career to create. An audience anticipates your talent. The only way to start is to start. Reach for the stars!

Wishing you every success,

Your success coach,

Cynthia Brian

Starstyle® Productions
PO Box 422
Moraga, Cal. 94556

About the Author

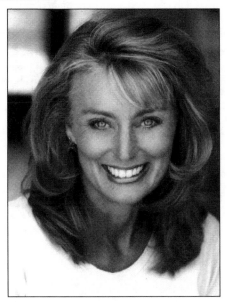

Cynthia Brian
Author, **The Business of Show Business**

Cynthia Brian, woman, wife, mother, actor, model, success coach, interior designer, gardener, artist, casting director, writer, New York Times best selling author, producer, world traveler, furniture designer, television and radio host...this lady is referred to as "the Renaissance Woman with Soul!"

Born on a farm in the Napa Valley in Northern California, the eldest of five children, she raised chickens and sheep, drove tractor and picked fruit to earn enough money to pay her way through college. After being named the Outstanding Teenager of California, she was named teenage ambassador to Holland where she studied for eighteen months while serving as foreign correspondent for several local newspapers and traveled throughout Europe. Thus began the world travels that would teach her to speak seven languages. Cynthia attended UCLA, the Universite de Bordeaux in France, and UC Berkeley, graduating with a B.A. in History.

Cynthia's passion for traveling and people is matched by her passion for acting which she has been doing professionally for over two and a half decades, working in films, commercials, and print ads with some of the biggest names in the entertainment industry. She has hosted several television shows and has been active in all phases of the acting world. Her company, Starstyle®

Productions offers private consultations on the business and her book The Business of Show Business has served as an extremely popular and useful guide. As an acting coach, she has guided the careers of several hosts for other talk shows as well as talent on established series.

Cynthia, a certified interior designer, is president of her own interior design firm, Starstyle® Interiors and Designs. Her designs have been featured in several books, magazines, newspapers and television shows. She produced A Gardener's Calendar and also designs furniture, including her popular Starstyle® Gametable and Ottomans.

She produces, writes and hosts two television series, Starstyle® Live Your Dreams, an inspirational program about people who are doing what they love in life; and Starstyle® The Business of Show Business, an educational program about how to get going and stay going while avoiding the scams in the entertainment industry. For three years she produced and hosted a weekly radio program interviewing best selling authors and was dubbed the "personal growth expert for business radio. As the Founder/CEO of the non-profit charity, Be the Star You Are®!, Cynthia is devoted to the distribution of positive programming while her charity empowers youth at risk through its library of books and other media. . Her literary accomplishments include being the co-author of the New York Times best seller, Chicken Soup for the Gardener's Soul (HCI), author of Be the Star You Are!®, 99 Gifts for Living, Loving, Laughing, and Learning to Make a Difference (Celestials Arts/Ten Speed Press) and author of the quote gift book, Magical Moments. With her teenage daughter, Cynthia co-hosted, Animal Cuts™ for radio and TV. Business Bytes™ is her internationally syndicated newspaper column and a popular radio segment . As a speaker, Cynthia presents keynote addresses on lifestyle, empowerment, gardening, and success issues around the country.

For a farm girl from Napa Valley, her hard work, enthusiasm, energy, action, and jamais di jamais (never say never) positive attitude have certainly added the sparkle to a starstyle life!

Contact info:
Cynthia Brian
Starstyle® Productions
PO Box 422
Moraga, California 94556
925-377-STAR (7827)
www.star-style.com
cynthia@star-style.com

Designated Charity

BE THE STAR YOU ARE®! EMPOWERS YOUTH!
(A portion of the proceeds from this book will be donated to this charity)

BE THE STAR YOU ARE®! Provides a Library of books and other media to empower youth at risk to improve their daily lives.

In 1997 juveniles under age 18 were involved in 27% of all serious violent victimizations, including 14% of sexual assaults, 30% of robberies, and 27% of aggravated assaults.

In 1998, nearly four in 10 fourth-graders nationwide failed to achieve even partial mastery of the reading skills needed for school success. In our highest-poverty schools, nearly seven in 10 fourth-graders fail to read at this Basic level.

Teens with poor self-esteem are more vulnerable to peer pressure, more likely to have depressive reactions, eating disorders, and low achievement standards. They are at higher risk to abuse alcohol and drugs, partake in violent activities, and to take risks such as driving dangerously.

BE THE STAR YOU ARE®! is a library of books and other media donated to youth at risk to raise their skills and self esteem to improve their daily lives. This media ranges from education and advisement to inspiration and guidance which covers every aspect of life from abuse through money management.

BE THE STAR YOU ARE®! has no religious or political agendas or affiliations as it caters to the literate and illiterate by providing audio tapes and videos as well as books to give these kids a head start in their lives so they can beat the odds.

BE THE STAR YOU ARE®! supplements the materials with a number of focused programs including Reading Spells Success! a literacy outreach program for young people. This program provides readers to children and teens to encourage and increase a literate younger generation.

BE THE STAR YOU ARE®! is actually saving trees as these donated books are mostly over runs, returns, early editions or slightly damaged books that were to be destroyed. Being a good steward of the earth is important to us.

A contribution to BE THE STAR YOU ARE®!, a volunteer organization, makes a difference in your community. Ask your company to match your donation.

BE THE STAR YOU ARE®! has seen the positive results these donations and programs make. We want to distribute more books and media as well as introduce more enrichment programs to help change the face of tomorrow from one of despair to one of hope for the next generation of adult citizens. All donations are 100% tax deductible and go directly to implement our mission. http://www.bethestaryouare.org

HOW YOU CAN HELP!

BE THE STAR YOU ARE®! believes that information infused with inspiration has the power to transform and change lives. BE THE STAR YOU ARE®! is a library of books and other media that empower youth at risk to improve their daily lives. BE THE STAR YOU ARE®! is committed to providing positive role models for kids to help them grow into valued citizens. Through its newsletters, web site, radio, TV, and READING SPELLS SUCCESS literacy outreach programs, BE THE STAR YOU ARE®! promotes and distributes its ever-growing list of informative positive videos, tapes and books to young audiences who would otherwise never obtain these materials. Recipients of BE THE STAR YOU ARE®! products and services include other non profit youth at risk groups, juvenile hall facilities, youth camps and children's hospitals.

In an era when violence and skepticism dominate the airwaves, BE THE STAR YOU ARE®! charity offers a refreshing, welcome alternative helping kids beat the odds encouraging the American Dream

Here are a few ways you can contribute:

v   Send a tax deductible contribution or offer a monetary tribute or memoriam to a loved one

v   Buy quantities of the three books which donate sales proceeds to our charity: **Chicken Soup for the Gardener's Soul** (HCI) and **Be the Star You Are! 99 Gifts for Living, Loving, Laughing and Learning to Make a Difference** (Ten Speed Press) and **The Business of Show Business** (Available through our office, on-line, or in stores)

v   Donate air miles

v   Donate goods that can be auctioned off at an event

v   Sponsor an event making BE THE STAR YOU ARE®! the charitable beneficiary

v   Ask your company to match your donation or make a contribution

v   Volunteer time

v   Become a Benefactor

v   Establish A Charitable Giving Account with an Investment Firm in the name of **BE THE STAR YOU ARE**®!.

Please join our galaxy of Stars and support BE THE STAR YOU ARE®! with your contributions and/or ask your company to be on our team.

For more information, call us at 925-376-7126 or 877-944-STAR. Send donations to: Be the Star You Are®! 501 (c) (3), PO Box 376, Moraga, California 94556.

Visit our web site at http://www.bethestaryouare.org for a free newsletter and news on special events. Get involved, make a difference, dare to care.

(Footnotes)
Adapted from Snyder, H. & Sickmund, M. Juvenile Offenders and Victims: 1999 National Report, p. 63. Washington, D.C.: Office of Juvenile Justice and Delinquency Prevention, 1999. Internet citation: OJJDP Statistical Briefing Book. Online. Available: http://www.ojjdp.ncjrs.org/ojstatbb/qa136.html. 30 September 1999.)

U.S. Department of Education, National Center for Education statistics. (1999). The 1998 NAEP Reading Report Card for the Nation. NCES 1999-459, by Donahue, P.L., Voelkl, K.E., Campbell, J.R., and

Mazzeo, J. Washington, D.C.: Author.

Article by Margaret S. Freidman, Psy D. "Parenting for self-esteem".

1997. http://www.coolware.com/health/medical_reporter/parent.html

Starstyle®

Starstyle® Productions, established in 1984, was originally Starstyle® Interiors because my belief was to "create beauty from the inside out" for all of my clients.

My purpose has always been process oriented, not product oriented so feeling one's soul or "interior" was essential. The focus of my work is teaching on-camera acting classes to children and providing consultations for parents and adults interested in getting into films and commercials. The format is to provide a safe, supportive environment where children can be themselves and feel that they are worthwhile individuals while pursuing an acting career. I empower children and their parents by providing them with the most updated honest information about this business and teach them survival techniques in this "starstruck" environment. Starstyle® Productions has expanded to include adults who want to get in touch with the child within, while providing casting services for producers and agents that benefit my clients, as well as private personal consultations and coaching.

I am a member of Screen Actors Guild, the American Federation of Television and Radio Artists, the National Academy of Television Arts and Science, Film Arts Foundation, and the National Association of Television Program Executives. The mantra of Starstyle® Productions is "Be the STAR you ARE!®"

Starstyle® Interiors and Designs draws on a successful career in film and television utilizing my artistic theatrical knowledge in residential decorative and design applications. The idea for interiors began with creating beauty from the inside out. I am a professional member of the American Society of Interior Designers, The Interior Design Society, California Council for Interior Design Certification, Allied Board of Trade as well as a NCIDQ certified interior designer. My design approach is to create exciting, dramatic designs that reflect the lifestyle and energy of my clients. The motto of Starstyle® Interiors and Designs is "Seeing the invisible to create the impossible...for the life You design!"

For more information on either Starstyle® Productions or Starstyle® Interiors and Designs, please check out our web site at:
http://www.star-style.com
or call 925-377-STAR to request a complimentary brochure.

Consultation and Coaching

Cynthia Brian's STARSTYLE®
CONSULTATIONS & ACTING COACHING:

"THE BUSINESS OF SHOW BUSINESS"

Cynthia Brian is a recognized expert in assisting talent enter the acting and modeling profession the right way while avoiding the scams. With over 26 years experience in all phases of the entertainment industry including acting, producing, writing, directing, coaching, and casting, Cynthia brings her unique qualifications and enthusiasm to a private consultation personalized to your specific needs. A consultation focuses on answering all your questions in an honest, no nonsense fashion, while creating a plan for your success. Coaching and consultations for all ages.

Most often asked questions are:

"How do I get started in acting and modeling?"

"Can I pay for college by doing this?"

"How do I get an agent?"

"How do I join the unions?"

"Do I need a portfolio?"

"Do I have the right look?"

"Will I need to move to Los Angeles of New York?"

"What kind of photographs do I need?"

"How can I recognize a scam?"

"Will I become a star?"

A private session will teach you the facts and myths about the entertainment industry and provide you with concrete tools to prepare you and your family for this business. Learn how to write an acting resume, a cover letter to agents, names and addresses of casting directors, agents, photographers, instructors, unions, printers, trade publications, and much much more. Buy the book The Business of Show Business for reference and more detailed information. A session is a MUST before spending time and money embarking on the journey to "the business of show business." Improve your communication skills and self-esteem.

To schedule your personal consultation, call Cynthia 925-377-STAR or email her cynthia@star-style.com.

Visit the website at http://www.star-style.com.

Cynthia Brian's STARSTYLE®

SUCCESS CONSULTATIONS & MEDIA COACHING

Cynthia Brian is a recognized expert in personal growth and achievement as well as a savvy marketeer. As the New York Times best selling author of Chicken Soup for the Gardener's Soul and the book, Be the Star You Are!, Cynthia has been a guest on over 500 radio and TV programs nationwide. She can help you change your life into the one you want to live and market yourself to the media. . With over 26 years experience in all phases of the entertainment industry including acting, producing, writing, directing,, coaching, hosting, and casting, as well as business in the design and garden industry, Cynthia brings her unique qualifications and enthusiasm to a private consultation and coaching session personalized to your specific success needs. Each session focuses on answering all your questions in an honest, no nonsense fashion, while creating a plan for your success in front of the media and in life. Coaching and consultations for all ages. Cynthia will custom tailor a group workshop for your group.

What you'll learn in a private media workshop:
☆ Learning to Breathe
☆ Body Language techniques
☆ How to think like a producer
☆ Creating a sound bite
☆ Pitching ideas and shows
☆ How to be in Show Business, whether you think you are or not!
☆ What to Wear to television and print interviews
☆ How to give a great interview without giving away family secrets
☆ How to avoid saying uhhh and sound intelligent on the air
☆ Getting the right head shot
☆ Creating hooks
☆ How to sound confident even if you aren't
☆ How to be a compelling guest that offers solutions
Most often asked career choice questions are:
☆ How can I discover my dream vocation?"
☆ Am I on the right track?"
☆ How can I do what I love and make a living?"
☆ What resources are available to help me?"
☆ Is my dream possible?"
☆ Do I need an agent or manager?"

☆ Will I need to move to another city?"

☆ How can I become a star?"

☆ How can I be successful and have a family?"

☆ How do I create support for my ideas?

A private session will guide you to discover your own gifts and talents and provide you with concrete tools to prepare you and your family for your new business. Improve your communication skills, self-esteem and confidence. Discover and learn more about YOU!

What Clients are saying:

"THANK YOU SO MUCH for all the good information and contacts you gave me at my media coaching session. My head is just filled with all of the things I can try now! Also thanks very much for the emails you've sent in advance of my contact. It will make a difference. You are truly an angel in my life!!! It's so nice to have someone who's already been there to help direct me and also keep me encouraged."

—Elisabeth Wilson, author of"*Kaleidoscope*

"You share a wealth of information and so freely. Your desire to help and inspire others comes from a deep within desire and you do it so well."

—Jean Kelly, author event coordinator, Barnes and Noble

"While being with you I got so many answers I was searching my heart for. You helped me so much. Things you said really opened my eyes and I thank you for that."

—Tami Rush, Greeting Card artist for Giant Smiles

Fees are on an hourly basis with a two hour minimum. Telephone or email consultations are also available. To schedule your personal consultation, call Cynthia at 925-377-STAR or email her cynthia@star-style.com.

Visit the website at http://www.star-style.com.

Order STARSTYLE® Products Directly

PRICE LIST

☆ Be the Star You Are! book	$15.95
☆ The Business of Show Business book	$19.95
☆ Miracle Moments® book	$ 9.99
☆ Chicken Soup for the Gardener's Soul book	$12.95
☆ Chicken Soup for the Gardener's Soul CD	$11.95
☆ Chicken Soup for the Gardener's Soul tape	$ 9.95
☆ Starstyle® Be the Star You Are! Radio tapes	$14.95

(visit Starstyle® Store web site for list)

☆ Special Reports (see web site for titles) $5.00- ea.

☆ PR Secrets of a Best Selling Author—

Video or Audio Cassette $29.95

☆ Video tapes of The Business of Show Business— $29.95 ea.

or SPECIAL OFFER (Save $135): $295.00 for all 14

Choose from:

1. Agents
2. Photographers
3. You've Got Photos, Now What?
4. Kids' Agents
5. Classes, Coaching, and Audtions
6. Casting Directors
7. Stunts and Stage Combat
8. Voice Overs
9. Managers and Teen Actors
10. Make Up and Hair
11. Protecting Our Children
12. Unions: SAG and AFTRA
13. SCAMS!
14. Tools of the Trade

Order form on following page.